AF669656

The Short Textbook of

Medical Helminthology

The Short Textbook of
Medical Helminthology

Satish Gupte MD
Professor and Head
Department of Microbiology
Gian Sagar Medical College and Hospital
Ram Nagar, Rajpura, Punjab, India

JAYPEE *The Health Sciences Publisher*

New Delhi | London | Philadelphia | Panama

Jaypee Brothers Medical Publishers (P) Ltd

Headquarters

Jaypee Brothers Medical Publishers (P) Ltd
4838/24, Ansari Road, Daryaganj
New Delhi 110 002, India
Phone: +91-11-43574357
Fax: +91-11-43574314
Email: jaypee@jaypeebrothers.com

Overseas Offices

J.P. Medical Ltd
83 Victoria Street, London
SW1H 0HW (UK)
Phone: +44 20 3170 8910
Fax: +44 (0)20 3008 6180
Email: info@jpmedpub.com

Jaypee-Highlights Medical Publishers Inc
City of Knowledge, Bld. 237, Clayton
Panama City, Panama
Phone: +1 507-301-0496
Fax: +1 507-301-0499
Email: cservice@jphmedical.com

Jaypee Medical Inc
The Bourse
111 South Independence Mall East
Suite 835, Philadelphia, PA 19106, USA
Phone: +1 267-519-9789
Email: jpmed.us@gmail.com

Jaypee Brothers Medical Publishers (P) Ltd
17/1-B Babar Road, Block-B, Shaymali
Mohammadpur, Dhaka-1207
Bangladesh
Mobile: +08801912003485
Email: jaypeedhaka@gmail.com

Jaypee Brothers Medical Publishers (P) Ltd
Bhotahity, Kathmandu, Nepal
Phone: +977-9741283608
Email: kathmandu@jaypeebrothers.com

Website: www.jaypeebrothers.com
Website: www.jaypeedigital.com

Managing Editor: Mrs Jyotsna Gupte

The Short Textbook of Medical Helminthology

First Edition: **2015**

ISBN 978-93-5152-617-9

Printed at Rajkamal Electric Press, Plot No. 2, Phase-IV, Kundli, Haryana.

PREFACE

Helminthiasis, especially filariasis and schistosomiasis are constantly posing health problems, especially in resource-limited populations. In spite of research work all over the world, helminthic infection control, treatment and preventon measures are not up to the mark.

Needless to add that complexity of problem has gained momentum because of unchecked population multiplication, poor socioeconomic conditions and poor sanitation, especially in developing countries. To add fuel to this crisis, we have so far failed to develop vaccines against helminths. Thus, helminths are having a field day to cause morbidity. However, a lot of work is in progress in this direction. Hopefully, in foreseeable future, we may get effective vaccine(s) against helminths.

Though helmiths are more prevalent in tropical countries, they have become a factor of concern all over the world in one way or the other. Sufferers include inhabitants of developed and developing countries, poor and rich alike. These worms have vital role to play in causing malnutrition, growth retardation, malignancy and what not.

The present book, *The Short Textbook of Medical Helminthology* aims at a comprehensive, reasonably illustrated and state-of-the-art update of helminths, a universal cause of morbidity and mortality.

Apart from routine worm description, the book provides discussion on such interesting topics as Emergence of Helminthic Infections, Helminthic Nosocomial Infection, Oncogenic Helminths, Control, Prevention and Vaccines, Treatment, etc. Hot topics like Schistosomiasis, Filariasis and Hydatidosis are discussed with up-to-date information. The book is adequately illustrated as well.

Hopefully this book with meaningful illustrations and up-to-date information shall be welcomed by the academicians and all those interested in helminths and allied issues.

I look forward to suggestions and constructive critical comments for bringing out improved future editions.

Satish Gupte

ACKNOWLEDGMENTS

At the very outset, I am grateful of M/s Jaypee Brothers for giving me the honor to pen down the book *The Short Textbook of Medical Helminthology*. In this regard my special thanks are due to Shri Jitendar P Vij, Group Chairman, for meaning cooperation and interaction from time to time in bringing out this volume within short time without compromising on production quality.

To the management and administration of Gian Sagar Medical College and Hospital, I respectfully take the opportunity to say "thank you".

I am thankful to my brother, Dr Suraj Gupte, Professor and Head, Postgraduate Department of Pediatrics, Mamta Medical College and Hospitals, Nellore, South India. In actuality, it was he who convinced me about the compelling need for such a book, assuring full help towards this assignment. He is a source of inspiration and role model for me.

My thanks are due to faculty members especially Dr Prerna Aggarwal, Dr Maninder, Dr Manju Bala, late Dr Ashok Kumar Chopra and Dr Ashwini Manhas of Microbiology Department, Gian Sagar Medical College and Hospital for critical constructive comments and for helping me to compile such topics as "Oncogenic Helminths, Emerging Helminthic Infections, and Control, Prevention and Vaccines and Treatment".

My gratitude to my wife and Managing Editor, Jyotsna Gupte, and son, Anubhav Gupte, for their contribution in various ways in the preparation of manuscript.

I am thankful to Mr Gurpreet Singh and Ms Kavita Arora for secretarial work and excellent typing of the manuscript in record time.

It is a pleasure to express my gratitude to Ms Preety Nagpal, Ms Rishu Sharma and Ms Puneet Kaur for furnishing the line illustrations.

CONTENTS

Introduction to Helminths 1

HELMINTHS

Helminth means worm (Greek helmins - worm). They are multicellular, bilaterally symmetrical, elongated, flat or round and three germ layered (triploblastic) metazoan. They are divisible into the following phyla.

1. *Phylum platyhelminthes:* They are flat, leaf-like or tape-like segmented, mostly hermaphrodite. Their alimentary canals incomplete or entirely absent and do not possess a body cavity. Human pathogenic helminths of this phylum are of two classes: the cestodes and the trematodes. They infact are the helminths of low organization.
2. *Phylum nemathelminthes*: They are elongated, cylindrical, unsegmented bodies with separate sexes, alimentary canal is complete and body cavity is very well present. There is no circulatory system. The body is of an outer layer of longitudinal muscles and a simple excretory system. They are better organized than platyhelminthes.

Table 1.1: Differences between cestodes, trematodes and nematodes

Features	*Cestodes*	*Trematodes*	*Nematodes*
Shape	Tape-like and segmented	Leaf-like and unsegmented	Elongated, rounded cylindrical and unsegmented
Sexes	Not separate	Not separate except in Schistosoma haematobium	Separate
Head end	Suckers usually with hooklets	Suckers without hooklets	Neither suckers, nor hooklets. Buccal capsule may be well developed
Alimentary canal	Absent	Present but incomplete with no anus	Present and complete with anus
Body cavity	Absent	Absent	Present
Examples	Tapeworms	Flukes	Roundworms

Top Helminths According to the WHO

- *Ascaris lumbricoides*
- Hookworms
- *Trichuris trichiura*
- Filarial worms
- Schistosomes.

Above mentioned helminths can even cause quite a number of deaths.

FEATURES OF HELMINTHS

- Helminths do not multiply in the body of humans. However, *Strongyloides stercoralis* and *Echinococcus granulosus* are exceptions.
- The outer layer or the tegument is quite tough. It may resist intestinal digestion of living worm.
- Helminths move by muscular contraction and relaxation. Suckers present in some helminths, may help in their movement. However, helminths have no special organs of movement.
- True body cavity is absent.
- In some helminths, the digestive system is either rudimentary or altogether absent. They get predigested nutrients from humans.
- The reproductive system is highly developed.
- The excretory system is just sufficient.
- The nervous system is quite primitive.
- Many helminths may need more than one intermediate host to complete their life cycle.
- Environmental factors, food habits, practices or customs, etc. influence and modify the transmission of helminthic diseases.
- Preparation of vaccine is difficult as helminths are multicellular.

FEATURES OF CESTODES

- They are dorsoventrally flattened, segmented and tape-like.
- Their size varies from a few millimeters to many meters.
- Habitat of adult worms is intestinal canal of the host.
- The body of adult worm comprises head (scolex), neck and strobilla.
- The strobilla contains a large number of proglottids (segments).
- Cestodes are hermaphrodite.
- Alimentary canal is absent.
- Excretory and nervous systems are present.
- Suckers (cup-like) are present on the scolex. Scolex may bear hooks and rostellum.
- Reproductive system is highly developed.
- Examples of cestodes are *Diphylobothrium latum, Echinococcus granulosus, Tenia solium, Tenia saginata and Hymenolepis nana.*

FEATURES OF TREMATODES

- They are dorsoventrally flattened like a leaf.
- They are also called fluke.
- They have segmented body which is covered with tegument.
- The size varies from 1mm to 3 cms sucker or more.
- They have two suckers: (a) anterior sucker also called oral sucker (b) posterior sucker with which parasite is attached to the host.
- Trematodes are hermaphrodite except schistosomes.
- Body cavity is not present.
- They lay eggs (oviparous).
- The alimentary tract is incomplete.

- The excretory system and nervous system are present.
- Reproductive system is highly developed.
- Eggs are operculated except in schistosomes.
- Examples are *Schistosoma haematobium, Paragonimus westermani, Fasciolopsis buski, Clonorchis sinensis*, etc.

FEATURES OF NEMATODES

- They are cylindrical and elongated which tapers at both ends.
- Sexes are separate and males are smaller than females.
- Size varies from 1 mm (*Trichinella spiralis*) in length to more than 1 m (*Dracunculus medinensis*).
- The cuticle is generally smooth. Striation, ridges, spines, bristles, etc. may be present which are utilized for the identification of worm.
- Alimentary canal is usually complete.
- In the body cavity, digestive, genital and other systems float.
- Circulatory system is absent.

SIGNIFICANCE OF NEMATODES

- More than a billion people are infected with one or more species of intestinal nematodes all over the world.
- They are more common in areas with poor faecal sanitation especially in developing countries.
- Nematodal infection may cause malnutrition and diminished working stamina. They are not fatal.
- Zoonotic nematodal infection do occur, e.g. trichostrongyliasis, capillarias abdominal angiostrongyliasis and anisakiasis.
- The life cycle is quite varied. *Strongyloides stercoralis* and *Enterobius vermicularis* may be transmitted from person to person. On the other hand, *Ascaris lumbricoides, Ancylostoma duodenale* and *Necator americanus* may have to pass through soil for development.
- Heavy burden of adult worms require repeated exposure to parasites in its infectious form (larva or egg). It needs so because helminths fail to replicate themselves. Hence, clinical diseases are seen only in those patients who are prolonged residents in endemic areas.
- IgE and eosinophilia in abnormal levels must prompt the clinicians to look for occult helminthiasis.
- It appears as if significant immunity to intestinal nematodes does not develop.

Helminthiasis—A Review

2

HISTORY OF HELMINTHS AND ASSOCIATED HELMINTH INFECTIONS

The history of helminths has been fascinating one and helminths have been the subject of excitement in medicine. Primitive tribes in Sarawak and North Borneo people could be aware of intestinal roundworm and tapeworms.[1] Quotations from the Bible clearly refer to helminth worms. Probably those who contributed to Bible were aware of existence of parasite worms. The Egyptian Papyrus Ebers (1500 BC) did refer to intestinal worms which bear the confirmation by discovering calcified helminths eggs in mummies dating from 1200 BC. Greeks especially Aristotle (384-322 BC) were aware of range of parasites in humans and animals. Greeks Roman physicians (Hippocrates 460-375 BC, Celsus 25 BC- AD 50 and Galen 129-200 AD) were aware of human roundworms (*Ascaris lumbricoides, Enterobius vermicularis* and tapeworms). Paulus Aegineta (625-690) describes very distinct *Ascaris, Enterobius* and tapeworm with good clinical description of disease they cause. Aviaenna an Arabic physician recognizes, *Ascaris, Enterobius vermicularis* and tapeworm. Dracunculus medinensis was also reported by him which was prevailing in Arab especially around Red sea.

There was very little contribution toward addition of literature regarding helminths in the Middle ages. Interesting many misconceptions erupted about helminths. Toothache and heart attacks were attributed to helminths.[1] Astonishingly chinese physicians thought that man must harbor three worms to be in good health. The notion and belief that worms were beneficial also extended into Europe.[2]

In 17th and 18th centuries, Linnaeus described 6 helminths worms, i.e. *Ascaris lumbricoides, Ascaris vermicularis* (i.e. *Enterobius vermicularis*), *Gordius medinensis* (i.e. *Dracunculus medinensis*), *Fasciola hepatica, Taenia solium* and *Taenia latum* (i.e. *Diphyllobothrium latum*).[3] Another three species were added to helminthic worms by 1782, i.e. *Trichuris trichiura, Taenia saginata* and *Echinococcus granulosus.* By 1845 *Trichinella spiralis* and *Loa loa* was added. Addition of *Ancylostoma duodenale, Schistonsona mansoni* and *Hymenolepis nana* was done by 1855. Between 1852 to 1890, *Strongyloides stercoralis, Wuchereria bancrofti Clonorchis sinensis, Fasciolopsis buski, Paragonimus westermani* and *Dipylidium caninum* were included.[4]

Almost 28 species had been recorded in human by the beginning of 20th century. The number became over 300 species.[5,6] Definitely with advances in biochemistry and molecular biology, there is creation of additional species and subspecies from within current list available.

Helminthic diseases contribute to mortality, morbidity, malnutrition, growth retardation and diminished work capacity. Adequate and reasonable knowledge of medical helminthology is desirable. Some of helminths diseases like onchocerciasis, soil transmitted nematodes, etc. are becoming public health problems especially in developing countries. Uprising of AIDS cases and other immunosuppressive conditions encourage opportunistic helminthic infections, e.g. strongyloidosis are attaining commanding positions all over the world including developed countries.

HELMINTHIC DISEASES BASED ON MODE OF INFECTION

1. **Contagious**: It is also called fecal or stool borne. Here infection may transmit directly from person-to-person, e.g. deposition of eggs at the anus, i.e. *Enterobius vermicularis*
2. **Soil transmitted**: Some eggs or larvae may require incubation in soil for sometime to become infective, e.g. *Ascaris lumbricoides, Ancylostoma duodenale, Necator americanus, Trichuris trichiura, Strongyloids stercoralis,* etc.
3. **Arthropod transmitted**: Arthopod is required as intermediate host for the development of infective stage in some helminths. It may transmit infection when bitten or eaten by human, e.g. *Wuchereria bancrofti, Brugia malayi, Dracunculus medinensis,* etc.
4. **Snail transmitted**: Small intermediate host allow the development of infective stages, e.g. schistosomiasis.
5. **Food animal transmitted**: In some animals infective stages of helminths develop. The flesh of these animals containing infective stages serve as item of food for humans, e.g. *Taenia solium, Taenia saginata,* etc.

PATHOGENIC ROLE OF HELMINTH

In fact it depends upon factors like number, habitat, pattern of laying eggs or larvae and products liberated from dead parasites. Helminths contribute towards pathogenesis as follows:

1. Physical obstruction, e.g. bunch of *Ascaris lumbricoides* may cause intestinal obstruction, perforation and necrosis. Even single roundworm may obstruct appendix or bile duct, thus causing appendicitis and obstructive jaundice, respectively. Obstruction of strongyloides to blood vessels may cause infraction.
2. Pressure effect, e.g. hydatid cyst exerts pressure producing damage to organ like eyes, brain, etc.
3. Lymphatic obstruction, e.g. *Wuchereria bancrofti* may cause elephantiasis because of repeated lymphangitis leading to lymphatic obstruction and lymphedema.
4. Trauma, e.g. *Ancylostoma duodenale,* etc. may cause, clinical disease of skin and intestine because of trauma .
5. Host reactions to parasites occur when parasites invade certain tissues of human body and there is excessive proliferation of the tissue, e.g. fibrosis or cirrhosis in liver due to deposition of ova of *Schistosoma mansoni* in the liver. The other example is hepatic fibrosis and hyperplasia of biliary epithelium in liver fluke infection (*Clonorchis sinensis* and *Fasciola hepatica*).
6. Tumor associated helminths may cause malignancy, e.g *Schistosoma haematobium* may contribute toward causing carcinoma urinary bladder. Likewise liver flukes like clonorchis and opisthorcis may have role in producing bile duct carcinoma. Cutaneous tumors were removed from a woman and they contained a coenurus (bladder worm) of multiceps serialis. Likewise tumor excised the intercostal muscle of northern Nigerian contained coemirus of multiceps glomeratus. There is also a report and incidence of *Hymenolepis nana* recovered from chest wall tumor of a 75-year-old Japanese woman.
7. By competing with host for food, *Diphyllobothrium latum* may cause B_{12} deficiency resulting in megaloblastic anemia.

8. Allergic syndromes, e.g. many dead helminths larvae release secretions and excretions producing allergic clinical conditions.
9. Evasion mechanisms, e.g. masking of antigen by schistosomes, suppression of immune response by *Trichinella spiralis, Schistosome mansoni,* sharing of antigen between parasite and host by schistosomes, there is continuous turnover plus release of surface antigens by schistosomes. With evasion mechanisms, helminths infact avoid elimination by host defence system.
10. Bacteria may contaminate the wound or ulcer produced by guinea worm.

Importance of helminthic disease: Helminthic diseases do occur worldwide especially in undeveloped tropical and sub-tropical areas. The factors responsible for wide prevalence of these diseases are high population density, poor sanitation deficient water source, poor personal hygiene, poverty and lack of resources etc. To worsen the situation environmental conditions prevail like deforesting, building of dams affecting breeding of vectors and density of reservoir host. To this list it is worth to add customs of local inhabitants.

Almost one-third of the world population is infected with helminths. Worldwide prevalence of some important helminths is as under:

Table 2.1: Worldwide prevalence of helminths

Diseases	*Parasites*	*Prevalence*
Ascariasis	*Ascaris lumbricoides*	100 crores
Hookworm diseases	*Ancylostoma duodenale* and *Necator americanus*	80 to 90 crores
Schistosomiasis	*Schistosome species*	20 to 30 crores
Filariasis	*Wuchereria bancrofti* *Brugia malayi, etc.*	25 crore
Pinworm infection	*Enterobius vermicularis*	5 to 10 crore
Guinea worm infection	*Dracunculus medinensis*	2 to 4 crore
Strongyloidiasis	*Strongyloides stercoralis*	5 to 8 crore

Of course these helminthic infections affect health, social and economic aspects of day-to-day life. Definitely these factors have role in malnutrition, growth retardation and diminished working stamina.

Sources of Infection

1. Contaminated soil and water usually mixed with human excreta provides source of infection of *Ascaris lumbricoides, Ancylostoma duodenale, Necator americanus, Strongyloides stercoralis* and *Trichuris trichiura*. The above mentioned parasites undergo development in the soil. They are named as soil transmitted helminths.

   On the other hand water contaminated with human excreta may have eggs of *Taenia solium, Hymenolepis nana,* and infective cercarial forms of *Schistosoma haematobium, Schistosoma mansoni* and *Schistosoma japonicum.*
2. Fresh water fishes may be responsible for making available source of *Diphyllobothrium latum* and *Clonorchis sinensis.*
3. Crab and cray fishes can be the sources of *Paragonimus westermani.*

4. Undercooked or raw pork may become the source of *Trichinella spiralis, Tenia solium,* etc.
5. Undercooked or raw beef can be the source of *Taenia saginata, Toxoplasma gondii.*
6. Water cress may provide source of *Fasciola hepatica.*
7. Blood sucking insect may spread Wuchereria bancrofti, Brugia malayi, Onchocerca vulvulus, etc.
8. Dog may act as a source of *Echinococcus granulosus, Toxocara canis,* etc.
9. Man can be a source of *Enterobius vermicularis, Hymenolepis nana,* etc.
10. Auto-infection may occur in case of *Enterobius vermicularis* and *Strongyloides stercoralis* resulting into hyperinfection.

Portal of Entry

1. *Mouth*: Through mouth helminths enter by contaminated food, water, soiled fingers or fomites, e.g. *Enterobius vermicularis, Trichuris trichiura, Ascaris lumbricoides, Trichinella spiralis, Taenia solium, Taenia saginata, Diphyllobothrium latum, Fasciola hepatica, Fasiolopsis buski, Clonorchis sinensis, Paragonimus westermani.*
2. *Skin*: Entry of this route by helminths is quite common, e.g. Ancylostoma duodenale, Necator americanus Strongyloides stercoralis, Schistosoma hematobium, Schistosoma mansoni, Schistosoma Japonicum, etc. Wucherchia bancrofti, Burgia malayi, Onchocerca volvulus, etc. are introduced when blood sucking arthopods puncture the skin to feed.
3. *Inhalation*: *Enterobius vermicularis* eggs might be inhaled into posterior pharynx.

WORLDWIDE STATUS OF HELMINTHS

Worm infection is a significant burden in Africans and other parts of the world.[7] Malaria and schistosomiasis cause highest burden all over the world. Intestinal worms produce the highest burden in children aged 5–14 years. Helminthic diseases may spread to other areas reaching new host through vectors, fecal contamination of soil, water, food and also through blood transfusion. Transfusion acquired helminthic infection include *Brugia malayi, Brugia bancrofti, Mansonella ozzardi, Mansonella perstans, Loa loa,* etc. However, this mode of transmission is quite rare even in endemic countries.

Food borne trematode such as opisthorchis species are responsible for diseases in migrants from South East Asia and the eastern Pacific High prevalence has been noticed in refugees in camps in Cambodia, Laos in Thai immigrant workers in Kuwait and China. Similarly pulmonary paragonimiasis is diagnosed in refugees from South East Asia residing in France and in the USA. Immigrants from Asia to Europe and USA[8] showed evidences of liver flukes. Ethiopian refugees in Israil harbor liver flukes too. The round worm and *Strongyloides stercoralis* are liable to be acquired by migrants and travelers to developing countries.

Dracunculiasis: Dracunculiasis occurs in around 16 sub-Saharan countries in Africa as well as in India and Pakistan. It involves ten African countries considered among least developed countries of the world. Worldwide cases reported in 1980s were 5–10 million which came down to 3 million in 1992, further declined to 229,773 in 1993 and to 164,973 in 1999. Around 2/3rd cases from Africa were contributed by Nigeria and Sudan.[9,10] In 1998 about 72000 cases were reported mainly from Ghana, Nigeria and Sudan.[11]

The success of eradication campaign is running in many countries being based on availability of potable water through the construction of safe and ideal wells and other preventive measures including boiling chlorination or filtration of water. Dracunculiasis eradication has been declared in India in 2000 by International Commission for certificate of Dracunaculasis Eradication.[12]

Filariasis: Around 90 billion people are infected with filariasis from 76 countries inhabitants living in endemic filariasis areas. Of these 72.8 million are infected with *Wuchereria bancroft* and 5.8 million from species of brugia.[9] There are 300,000 cases of filariae in seven countries in Americas, 48.6 million in South East Asia, 3.9 million in 14 countries of Western Pacific and 25.6 million in 40 countries in Africa.[13] About 40 million persons worldwide suffer from lymphedema elephantiasis or hydrocele caused by bancroftian filariasis. Worldwide brugia is believed to cause lymphedema, elephantiasis in 208 million of whom 1900,000 are in South East Asia and 900,000 are in Western Pacific (WHO).

In India infected person suffer 4.47 acute attacks per year if they suffer from bancroftian filariasis and 2.20 acute attacks per year if they have brugian filarasis. Each attack has an average duration of 4 days and number of working days wasted per year are 1743 and 891 for bancroftian and brugian filariasis respectively.[13] Almost 75 and 122.9 million persons are at risk of onchocerciasis (river blindness) which remains endemic in 28 countries in Africa and 6 countries in America. In Africa 17.7 million persons are infected with Onchocerca volvulus of whom 500,000 have damaged vision and 267,000 are blind. In America 140,000 people are infected with onchocerciasis of whom 750 are blind.[15]

Filariasis is caused by vector borne tissue dewelling nematodes called filariae. Adult may live in lymphatics, blood vessels, skin connective tissues or serous membranes depending upon species of worm involved. Microfilariae are liberated by female adult worm. The microfilariae may live in bloodstream or skin. All true filariae causing infection in humans, e.g. Onchocercidae are transmitted by dipterm vector. The transmission of human filariae is mostly limited to warm climate. High temperature is necessary for parasite to develop in vector

The infective form of the parasite is third stage larvae which may be transmitted by vector. The rate of growth, life cycle, differentiation of worms, longevity of microfilariae and adult worms differ widely between different species. The life span of some adult worm may extend upto 20 years even.

Onchocerciasis and lymphatic filariasis are quite significant infections dracunculiasis may cause ulceration and calabar swellings. Loasis may result to other manifestation leading to severe consequences to the patients.

FOOD BORNE TREMATODE INFECTIONS

Human disease may be caused by trematode likes fasciola, opisthorchis, clonorchis, paragonimus, and fasciolopsis, etc. *Opisthorchis felineus* is usually acquired by eating raw frozen fish in Siberia.

Effects to control food borne trematodes are revolutionized by the drug praziquantel. Other factors involved to control, this condition includes improvement in sanitation and health promotion to encourage proper cooking of foods involved in transmission.

HELMINTHS OF EYE IMPORTANCE

1. *Echinococcus granulosus.*
2. *Taenia solium.*
3. *Fasciola hepatica.*
4. Larva of *Ascaris lumbricoides.*
5. Microfilariae of *Onchocerca volvulus* may cause corneal opacity, keratitis, iridocyclites and secondary glaucoma. As a result patient may develop irreversible damage of optic nerve leading ultimately to blindness.
6. The migrating adult worm of *Loa loa* are troublesome while passing in front of the eye ball. Further they have been removed from eyelids, anterior chamber of the eye and the bulba conjunctiva.
7. *Dracunculus medinensis* was removed from sub-conjunctival space of the eye of an Indian patient.

HELMINTHS OF CARDIAC IMPORTANCE

1. *Taenia solium* (Cysticercus cellulosae) may produce myocarditis or congestive heart failure.
2. *Echinococcus granulosus* may develop on the heart valves.
3. *Clonorchis sinensis* may produce symptoms of palpitation of the heart and tachycardia.
4. *Trichinella spiralis* may produce hypotension myocarditis and so on.
5. *Strongyloides stercoralis* may be found in heart.
6. Larvae of *Toxocara* canis and *Toxocara catis* may cause cardiac dysfunction.
7. *Ancylostoma duodenal* infection might produce palpitation of the heart the signs of high output and congestive heart failure.
8. A wondering worm of *Ascaris lumbricoides* may invade heart.

HELMINTHS OF GYNECOLOGICAL IMPORTANCE

1. Arthropod borne teniasis
2. Arthropod borne helminthic diseases:
   a. Filariasis (Culex, Aedes, Anopheles mosquito).
   b. Onchocerciasis (Simulium black fly).
   c. Mansonelliasis ozzardi (Culicoides furens).
   d. Loaiasis (Chrysops dimidiate, mango fly).
   e. Drancunculosis (Diaptomus, Cyclops).

EMERGENCIES AND HELMINTHIASIS

Abdominal pain and other discomfort are quite common to heavy small intestinal nematodes infections especially ancylostomiasis and *Ascaris lumbricoides.*[16] Anisakiasis which is acquired by eating undercooked or raw infected fish (sushi etc.) and the patient may present with acute appendicitis.[17,18] The disease above mentioned is invasive involving ileocecal area. It cannot be diagnosed satisfactory parasitologically or by undertaking serology test. This condition is not effective by chemotheraphy. For this only diagnostic laparotomy is required.

A disease called eosinophilic enteritis of multiple etiology[19] is prevailing. In a report a dog hookworm (*Ancylostoma caninum*) was found for an epidemic comprising of 93 cases.[20]

A rare case of acute mesenteric ischemia caused by *Schistosoma mansoni* has been reported from Baghdad (Iraq).[21] However, the small intestine may be involved in *Schistosoma japonicum* infection. Intestinal obstruction because of mesenteric ischemia may lead to intussuscepting polypoid mass or fibrotic stenosis. Intestinal perforation because of acanthocephalan worm (*Macracanthohynchus hirudinaceus*) a natural parasite of pig has been described in Bangkok, Thailand.[22] This infection is also reported from several other ports of the world, e.g. China, Southern Europe, etc.

Fatal gastrointestinal hemorrhage associated with fluctuating Jaundice, a tender liver, palpable gallbladder and eosinophilia is attributed to liver fluke *(Fasciola hepatica)* infection.[23] The site of bleeding was perhaps biliary tree.

REFERENCES

1. Hoeppli, R. Parasites and parasitic infection in early science and medicine: Singapore University of Malaya Press 1959.
2. Foster, WD. A history of parasitology. Edinburgh: Livingstone 1965.
3. Linnaeus, C. Systema Naturae, sive regina triae naturae systematice proposita por classes, ordines, genera, species cum characteribus1758.
4. Grove DL. A history of helminthology. Wallingford CAB International 1990.
5. Coombs. I and Crompton, DWT. A guide to human helminthology London: Taylor and Francis 1991.
6. Ashford, RW and Crewe W. The parasites of Homo sapiens, 2nd Edn. London: Taylor and Francis 2003.
7. World Bank Investing in Health. Development indicators. World Development Report 1993b. Oxford. Oxford University Press. 1993b; 213-25.
8. WHO, control of food borne trematode infections, WHO Tech Rep Ser 849. Geneva: World Health Organization 1995b.
9. WHO, Global Health Situation IV. Selected Infection and parasitic diseases due to identified organisms. WHO Wkly Epidemiol Rec, 1993C;680:43-44.
10. WHO Dracunculiasis. WHO, Wkly Epidemiol Rec. 1995C:70:125-32.
11. WHO, Report on infectious diseases removing obstacles to healthy development. Geneva, World Health Organization 1999.
12. Gupte, The Short Textbook of Medical Microbiology, 2006.
13. WHO, Lymphatic filariasis: The disease and its control, WHO, Tech Rep Sec 821. Geneva: World Health Organization 1992b.
14. WHO, Control of tropical diseases I. Progress report WHO CTD/MIP/94.4 Geneva: World Health Organization, 1994f:27-31.
15. WHO Onchocercosis and its control: WHO Tech Rep Sec 852, Geneva: World Health Organization 1995d.
16. Raj SM, Sivakamaran S, Vijay Kumari S. Morbidity due to intestinal helminthiasis. Lancet 1990:336:811-12.
17. Adams AA, Bech JL, Wekell MM. Health risk of salmon, sushi. Lancet 1990:336;1328.
18. Cook GC. Parasitic Disease in Clinical Practice: Springer, 1990;272.
19. Hepburn NC. Aetiology of eosinophilic enteritis. Lancet 1990;336.
20. Prociv and Croese J. Human eosinophilic enteritis caused by dog hookworm *Ancylostoma caninum*. Lancet 1990;335:1299-1302.
21. Anyi S and Al Nasiri N. Acute mesenteric ischemia caused by *Schistosoma mansoni* infection. BMJ 1987:294:294–1197.
22. Radomyos P, Chobchuanchom A, Tungtrongechitr A. Intestinal perforation due to Macracan Thorhynchus hirudinaceus infection in Thailand. Trop. Med. Parasitol 1989;40:476–77.
23. Bannerman C and Manzur AY. Fluctuating Jaundice and intestinal bleeding in 6-year-old girl with fasciolilasis. Trop Geogr Med 1986;38:429–31.

Intestinal Helminths 3

TRICHINELLA SPIRALIS

Synonyms

Trichina worm.

Discovery

- The disease trichinellosis was first of all described by Tidemann in Germany in 1821.
- Peacock and Owen from London reported this disease in 1835.
- Larval stage of *Trichinella spiralis* was demonstrated in human blood in 1909 by Herrick and Janewly.

Geographical Distribution

- It is cosmopolitan disease.
- It is predominantly found in Europe and America.
- It is not prevalent as a human disease in Africa and India.
- One human case was reported from Punjab (India) in 1996.

Habitat

It is an intestinal parasite. It remains buried in the mucosa of duodenum and jejunum where adult worms are found. Female fertilized adult worm discharges embryo into circulating blood which get encysted in striated muscles of host, e.g. pig, rat, man, etc.

Morphology

- It exists as adult form and larval form.
- Adult males are 1.4 to 1.6 mm long.
- Adult female are 4 mm long.
- Females are viviparous.
- Larvae measures 0.5 mm × 0.2 mm which contain 1 mm long coiled larva. Encysted larvae live longitudinally along the striated muscle fibers.
- Each female produces 1000 to 1500 larvae in its life span of 5–7 weeks.
- Larvae are passed in the stools.

Life Cycle

- The life cycle is passed in one host only (man, pig or rat).
- The primary host is pig which acts as reservoir host for man.
- Man is dead end for the parasite.

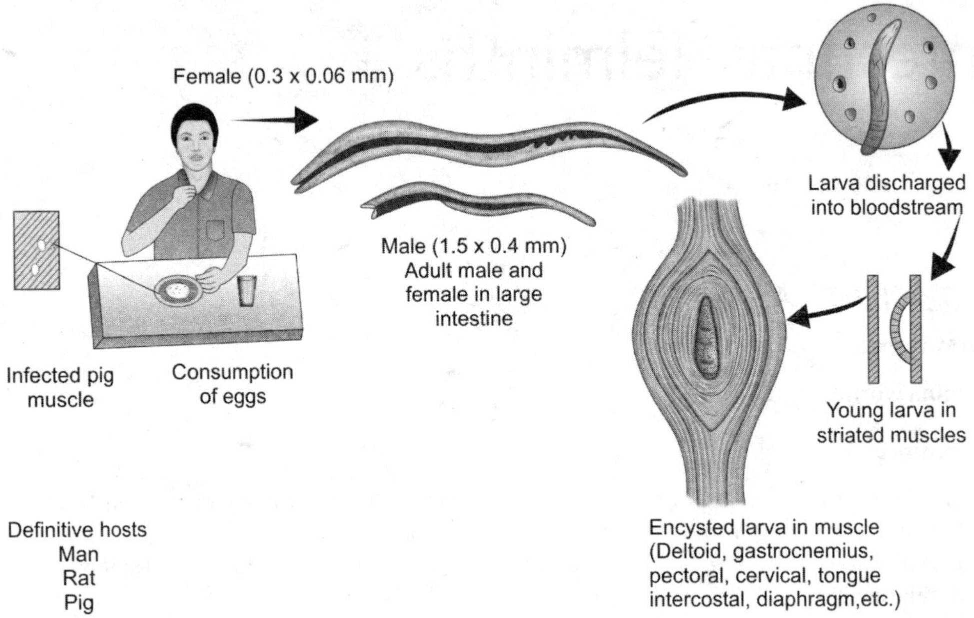

Fig. 3.1: Pathogenesis of *Trichinella spiralis*

- Transference of host is obligatory for continuation of race.
- After ingestion of infected meat the capsule of encysted larva is digested by gastric secretion, thus releasing larva in duodenum and jejunum.
- The newborn larva migrates from the small intestine to the muscle tissue via lymphatic circulation and blood stream invading tissues. The stage is most pathogenic form of parasite.[1]
- Four moultings occur in duodenum and jejunum, and larvae develop into adult forms.
- Male worm dies after mating female worm.
- Female worm get fertilized and deliver embryos, after 4–7 days of infection. The larvae after penetration of intestinal wall migrate through lymphatic vessels to blood stream taking them to various organs of the body.
- Larvae survive in skeletal muscles.
- During 3rd and 4th week of infection larvae develop in muscles.
- Larvae grow 10 times from 1 mm initial size.
- Cysts develop in muscles.
- Cysts usually occur at the insertion of muscles.
- The heavily affected muscles are diaphragm, intercostal, pectoral, tongue, muscles of jaw and extraocular.
- Deltoid musle is selected for the purpose of taking biopsy.
- There are three principal maintenance cycles, i.e.
  - Pig to pig
  - Rat to rat
  - Sylvatic, perpetuated by carnivorous wild hosts

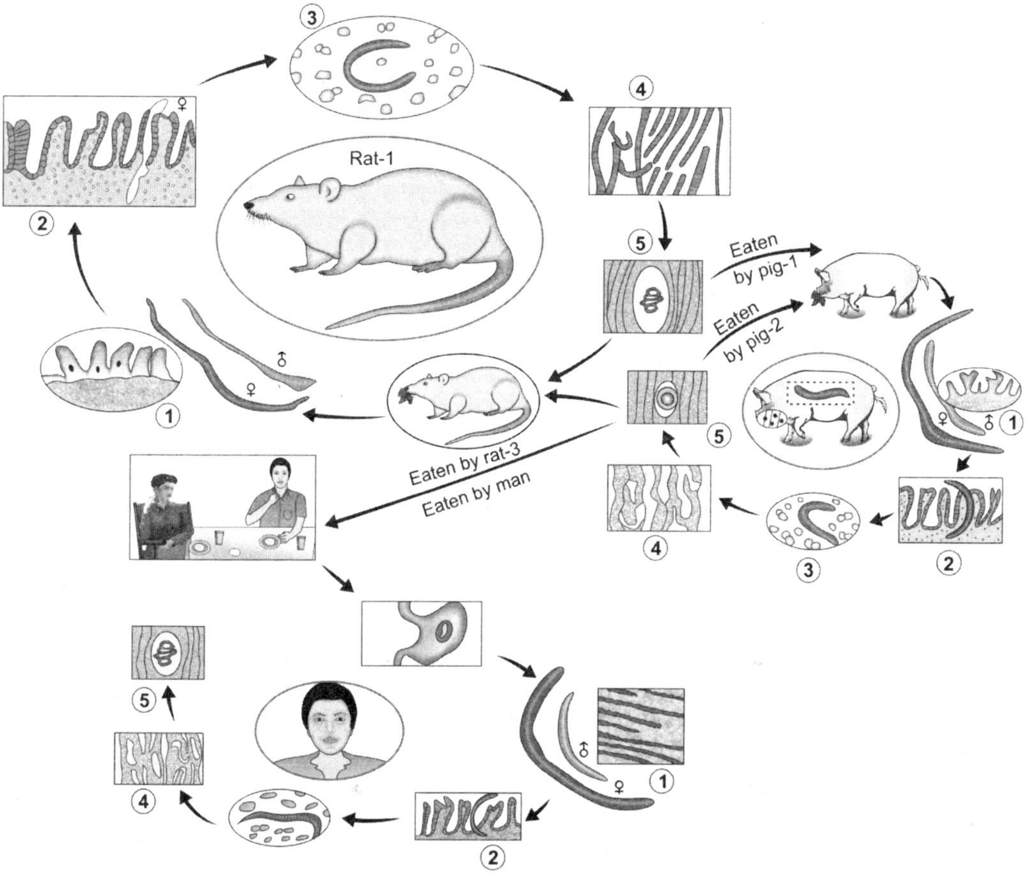

Fig. 3.2: Life cycle of *Trichinella spiralis*

Pathology

- At the site of adherence of adult worm the mucosa becomes hyperemic with potential hemorrhage.
- Important pathologic changes occur because of presence of larvae in the muscles.
- Larvae may invade myocardium.
- Myocardium becomes soft and flabby with fatty degeneration.
- In lungs there occurs edema, hemorrhage and eosinophilic abscess indicating allergic responses.
- In brain matter edema, hyperemia, punctate hemorrhage may occur with microscopic nodules.
- Larvae are found in cerebrospinal fluid and meninges.
- In case of decomposition of muscle cyst may remain viable for 10 days.

Clinical Features

- Light infections are asymptomatic.
- Manifestations of enteric phase include pain in abdomen, nausea, vomiting and diarrhea.

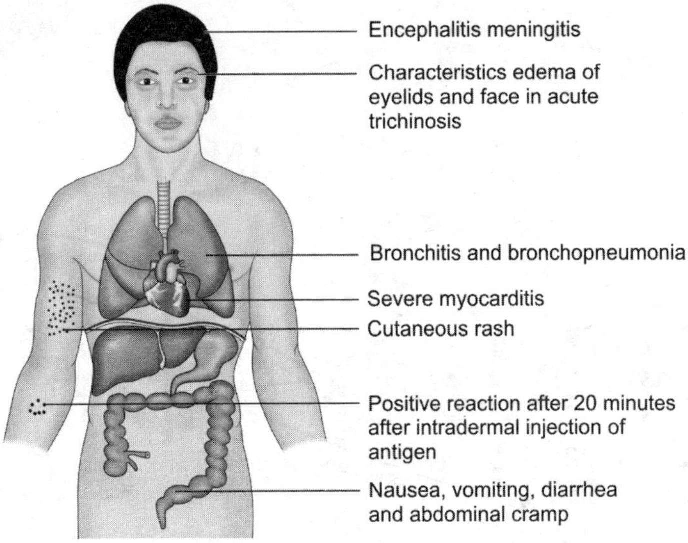

Fig. 3.3: Clinical features of *Trichinella spiralis*

- During larval migration hypersensitivity reactions occur, e.g. fever eosinophilia, periorbital edema, facial edema splinter hemorrhages, etc.
- In heavy infection (more than 50 larvae per gram of muscle), fatal myocarditis, encephatitis, pneumonitis, etc. may occur during larval migration only.
- The phase of larval migration may be asymptomatic in light infection (less than 10 larvae per gram) of muscle.
- In symptomatic case the patients may have manifestations of myalgia and weakness.

Laboratory Diagnosis

1. **DLC**: It shows significant eosinophilia upto 50–70%
2. **Muscle enzymes**: Due to attack of larvae on muscle there is elevation of muscle enzyme, e.g. lactate dehydrogenase, aldolase and creatnine phosphokinase.
3. **Muscle biopsy**:
   - Ideally it is done after 4th week of infection
   - A sample of one gram of muscles (biceps or gastrocnemius) is excised
   - Muscle sample collected is divided into two parts one is examined unstained while other one is stained
   - In moderate infection 50–100 larvae per gram of biopsy material are present
   - More oftenly 5000 larvae per gram of tongue biopsy material have been observed.
4. **Muscle digestion**
   - Muscle digestion is done for 30 minutes in 2% pepsin in saline containing 5% hydrochloric acid at 37°C
   - Now larvae are observed under the microscope. This method may be used for epidemiological purposes to assess the prevalence of larvae.
5. **Xenodiagnosis**: The biopsy material is fed to rats. After killing rats in around one month, larvae may be demonstrated in the muscles of rat.

6. **Skin test**: Brachman's antigen is used in 1:10,000 dilutions. This antigen is prepared using infected rabbit muscles. In positive case erythematous rash occurs within 15–20 minutes. However positive test remains positive upto 20 year.

Apart from above mentioned test larvae may be detected in blood, cerebrospinal fluid, etc. Some serological tests may be used like bentonite flocculation test (significant titer 1:5), indirect fluorescent antibody test, etc. These test cross react with salmonella.

Treatment

- Thiabendazole in doses of 50 mg/kg body weight per day for 5–7 days is very effective against migrating larvae and to some extent encapsulated forms also
- Pyrantel pamoate may be used against intestinal infection
- For intestinal infection tetramisole may be administered
- In addition prednisolone (1 mg/kg body weight) can be given in severe myositis and myocarditis.

Preventive Measures

- Eating meat is the typical way of acquiring infection with Trichinella spiralis.[2] One needs to be careful
- Proper cooking of pork. Larvae in porks are killed by heating above 55°C and may prevent human infection
- Proper storage by freezing pork at -15°C for 3 weeks is sufficient and safe for consumption
- Feeding of pigs with raw garbage must be avoided.

TRICHURIS TRICHIURA

Synonyms

Whip worm.

Discovery

- First discovered by Linnaeus 1771
- Later important contribution in understanding this infection was added by Schrank 1768 and Stite 1901.

Geographical Distribution

- It is the third commonest nematode after roundworm and hookworm to infect man.
- About 50 crore persons are infected worldwide
- It is common in moist and warm areas like South East Asia, Caribbean and tropical Africa
- Its distribution is restricted as its eggs are less resistant to environmental stress, e.g. drying and exposure to sunlight
- Interestingly the infestation of the *Trichuris trichiura* is most common but actually disease occurs in quite less number.

Habitat

The adult worm lives in cecum and appendix of man. However in heavy infections, the organisms are present all over the length of large intestine.

Morphology

Adult Worm

- They are pinkish white.
- The male worm is 30 to 40 mm long with coiled posterior end single spicule.
- The caudal end of male worm is curved ventrally.
- The female worm is slightly longer, i.e. 40 to 50 mm with posterior end straight, blunt and rounded.
- Both sexes have narrow and thin anterior portion (3/5th) and wider posterior end (2/5th). Hence called whip worm.
- The anterior thin portion containing capillary esophagus remains buried in the intestinal mucosa of host. The intestine and reproductive organs are located in the posterior thick part of the body.
- The female worm is oviparfsous.

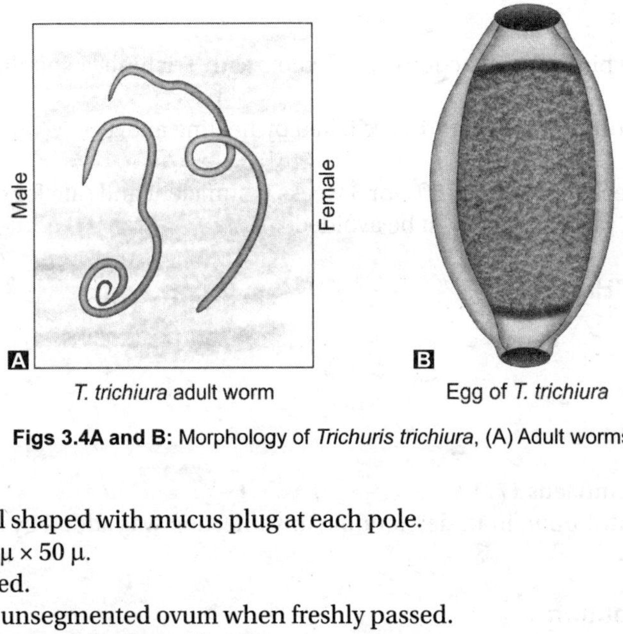

Figs 3.4A and B: Morphology of *Trichuris trichiura*, (A) Adult worms, (B) Eggs

Eggs

- It is barrel shaped with mucus plug at each pole.
- Size is 25 μ × 50 μ.
- Bile stained.
- Contains unsegmented ovum when freshly passed.
- Floats in saturated saline solution.
- The female worm may lays about 2000 to 10,000 eggs per day.

Life Cycle

- Life cycle takes place in one host only and change of host is required to continue new life cycle
- Eggs take 3 weeks to develop in moist soil and remain infective for 2 weeks. If the climate is temperate it may take 10–12 months. In dry condition embryonation may be prevented
- On ingestion of embryonated eggs with food and water, the shell of eggs may be digested by digestive secretions and lavae are liberated through one pole
- Larvae liberated are migrated to cecum

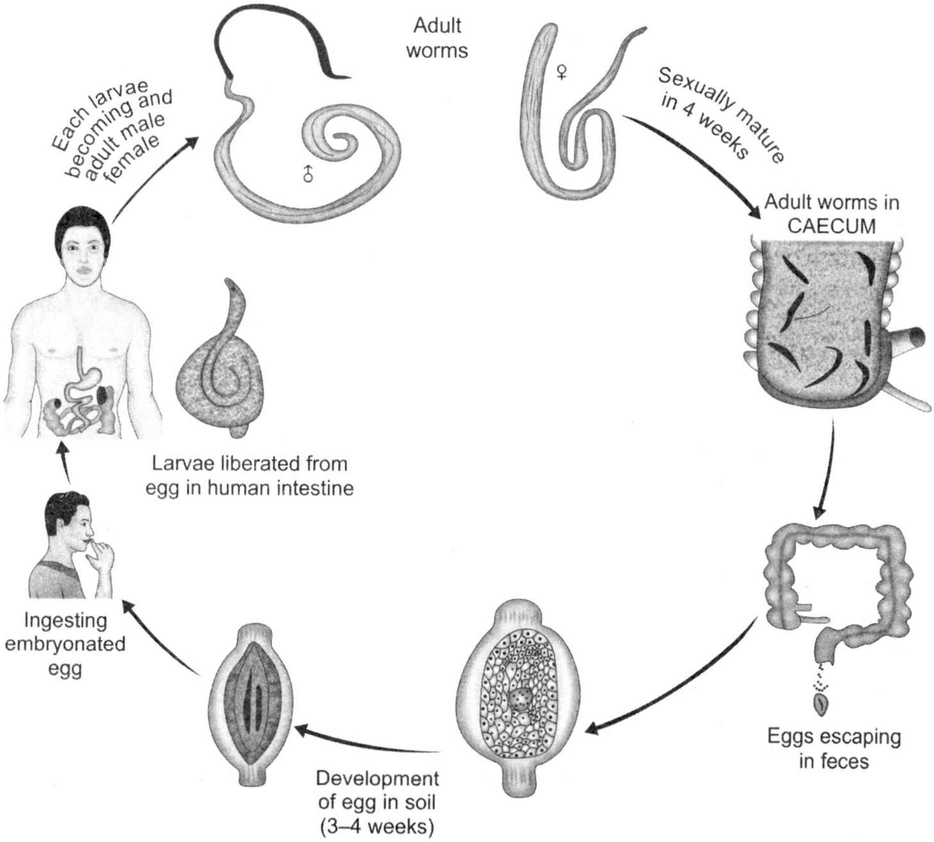

Fig. 3.5: Life cycle of *Trichuris trichiura*

- In cecum anterior thin portion gets embedded in the mucosa and posterior end hangs free projecting in the lumen of intestine. They develop into adult form and differentiate into males and females. Male fertilizes female.
- Egg starts appearing in stools usually in 3 months after ingestion of infective eggs. These eggs develop to infective form in the soil and hence infective to new host.
- The adult worms normally live for about 3 years but may survive upto 8 years.

Pathogenesis

- Anterior portion of worm embedded in the mucosa of intestine may cause petechial hemorrhages which may predispose the patients to infections with *Entameba histolytica* and *Shigella* species.
- The degree of inflammation may extend from the disital part of small intestine to rectum depending on the intensity of infection.[3]
- Entry of parasites in the lumen of the appendix may cause appendicitis or granuloma formation.

Clinical Features

- *Trichuris trichiura* causes trichuriasis
- Light *Trichuris trichiura* infections are asymptomatic
- Heavy infections are highlighted as
  - Abdominal pain
  - Children having infection with this parasite often suffer from chronic dysentry[4]
  - Rectal prolapse is due to toxic irritation of nerve endings. Mechanism of prolapse is similar to that of intussusception. Remission often occurs within few days of effective anthelminthic chemotherapy
  - Anemia due to heavy worm load (blood loss is 0.005 ml per worm)
  - Malnutrition
  - Bloody diarrhea
  - Ingestion of non-food substances, e.g. soil
  - Acute appendicitis (mechanical blockage)
  - Reversible clubbing of fingers in children, because of congestive heart failure secondary to severe anemia.

Laboratory Diagnosis

- DLC: It shows eosinophilia
- Stool examination: It shows
  - Charcoal Leydon crystals
  - Typically barrel shaped eggs
  - About 20,000 egg per gram are likely to produce clinical disease
- Sigmoidoscopy: In heavy infections it may show white bodies of worm hanging.

Pathology

- Immature *Trichuris trichiura* buries its entire body in the epithelium of large intestine constituting a tunnel.
- With the maturation of worm, the posterior part is extruded or get ruptured from tunnel, hangs in the lumen of intestine and becomes available for copulation and ovipositions.
- The intimate contact of *Trichuris trichiura* with the mucosa of large intestine causes inflammation and petechial hemorrhages of mucosa which may extend from the distal part of intestine right upto rectum. The mucosa may be edematous and friable.
- Rectal prolapse may occur as a result of strain to defecate.
- Rectal bleeding with abdominal cramps may occur with servere rectal tenesmus in case of massive infection.
- Massive infection may lead to iron deficiency anemia because of malnutrition and blood loss from friable colon and prolapsed rectum. The reaction with inflamed mucosa called coconut cake rectum.

Treatment

- Albendazole : 400 mg single dose
- Mebendazole : 100 mg in mild or moderate infection
  However heavy infection require 3 days treatment
- Oxantale : 20 mg/kg body weight for two consecutive days is highly effective

Prophylaxis

- Proper disposal of human excreta
- Use of solution of chloropicrin to kill eggs of this worm in soil
- Not to eat raw or uncooked vegetables and unwashed fruits
- Treatment of infected persons.

STRONGYLOIDES STERCORALIS

Synonyms

Anguillula stercoralis.

History

- Normand in 1876 identified strongyloides first of all in stools of French troops suffering from cochin - China Diarrhea.

Geographical Distribution

- This worm is widely distributed in Africa, Asia and South America
- It is found sporadically in North America and Europe.

Habitat

After getting fertilized adult female lives buried within the mucosa of small intestine particularly duodenum and jejunum.

Morphology

It occurs in adult form and larval form. It may be parasitic in nature or free living.

Parasitic Adult Form

- Males adult have not been seen in humans
- Males cannot penetrate intestinal wall and so they are immediately expelled by bowel by the time females start laying eggs
- Female adults live within mucosa of small intestine
- Female adult measures 2.5 mm × 0.04 to 0.05 mm
- It bears small buccal cavity surrounded by four lips
- It has two uteri filled with 10 to 20 eggs at a time
- It is ovo-viviparous. The eggs are thin shelled about 25 μ × 30 μ in dimension
- The eggs are laid in tissue.

Free Living Adults

- They live in moist soil
- Female is 1 mm long and males measure 0.7 mm long
- They mate in soil
- The fertilized females lay eggs that develop to rhabditiform larva

Larva

- Rhabditiform larva comes out of eggs and makes its way into lumen of intestine.
- Rhabdiliform larvae (200 to 300 μ × 16 μ) are expelled with feces. The larvae are actively motile.
- The larval bear small mouth and characteristic double bulb esophagus.

Life Cycle

- *Strongyloides stercoralis* complete the life cycle in one host.
- Man contacts this infection following contact with fecally contaminated soil or by autoinfection.
- Rhabiditiform larvae develop into filariform larvae in the soil.
- Flariform larvae are the infectious form that penetrate intact skin or mucus membranes
- After penetration larvae pass through blood stream enter lungs where they break into alveli, ascend bronchial tree, crawl over epiglottis and are swallowed down to small intestine. Here they develop and mature to adult form.
- Now female worm sheds eggs either by parthenogenesis or after fertilization by male worm
- Eggs develop locally in intestinal mucosa to release rhabdilitiform larvae which ultimately move into intestinal lumen.

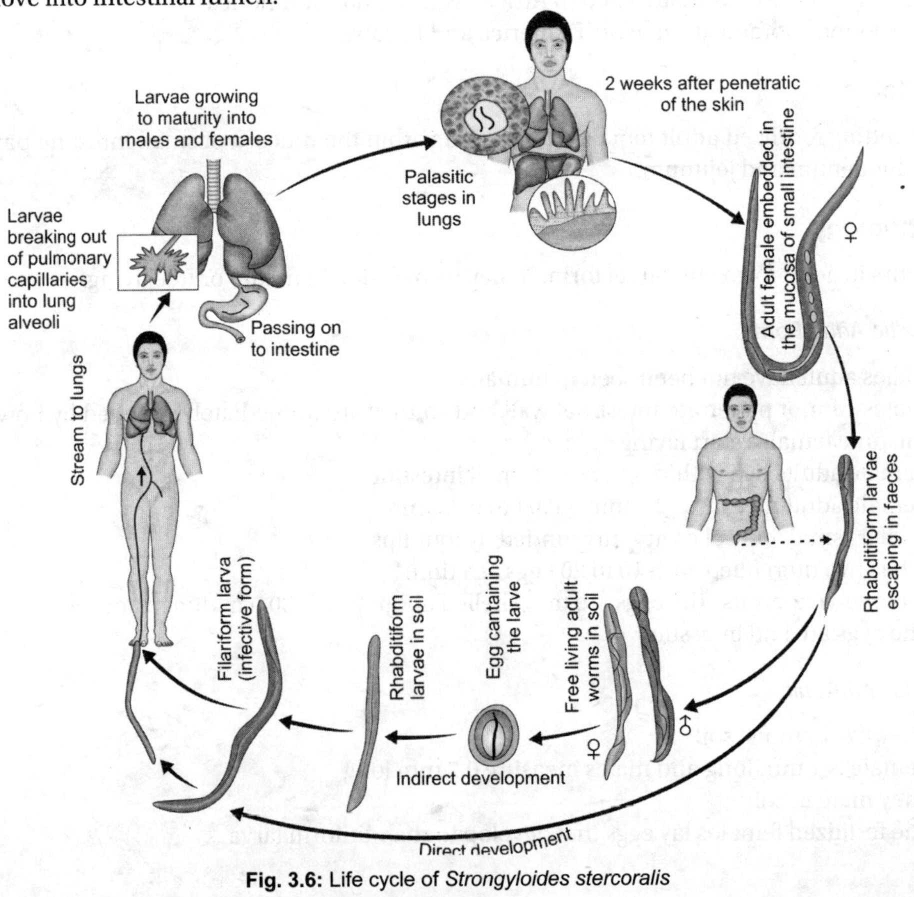

Fig. 3.6: Life cycle of *Strongyloides stercoralis*

- The rhabditiform larvae either pass with feces to the soil or develop to filariform larvae in the lumen of intestine
- The filariform larval may result to auto infection by penetrating mucosa or perianal skin
- Rhabiditiform larvae expelled with feces into the soil develop in two ways:
  - They mature to infective form i.e. filariform larvae
  - They may transform into free living adult males and females. The male worm fertilized female worm. The gravid female sheds eggs in soil which grow to filariform larvae. Filariform larvae penetrate the skin of new human to continue the cycle.

Pathogenesis

Infection caused by it is called strongyloidiasis. It may involve skin. The pathognomonic cutaneous symptoms of stongyloidiasis is larvae currens migrating larval produces raised erythematous lesion that moves along the course of migration larva currens also called running larva. It may move at 10 cm per hour. Migrating larvae may also produce hemorrhagic lesions in lungs. Burrowing adult worm may cause mild epigastric pain, gastrointestinal bleeding, mild chronic colitis, etc.

Conditions favouring suppressed or lowered immune status are immunosuppressive treatment, malignanacy, malnutrition, pregnancy, AIDS, etc. In this situation *Strongyloides stercoralis* infection results into hyperinfection. Large number of filariform larvae invade gastrointestinal tissues resulting to colitis, steatorrhea and dehydration. The larvae may harm CNS, peritoneum liver and kidneys, etc.

Several complication may occur because of bacteria from intestine which may enter through mucosa broken by penetrating larvae. These complications include septicemia, pneumonia, meningitis, etc.

Clinical Features

- Chronic infection with this parasite is most oftenly asymptomatic[5]
- There may be abdominal pain, nausea, vomiting, weight loss, gastrointestinal bleeding, pruritis, etc. These are acute manifestations
- Chronic manifestations include paralytic ileus and protein losing enteropathy, etc.
- Other presentations may be rash, meningitis, bronchopneumoniae and so on.

Laboratory Diagnosis

1. Demonstration of eggs, rhabditiform larvae, filariform larvae and adult female worm in papnicolou stained smear of stools, sputum or duodenal aspirate.
2. Repeated stool examination, aspiration of duodenal jejunal contents, biopsy or Entero test method may be used to improve detection rate of *Strongyloides stercoralis.*
3. Concentration techniques for stool examination may be tried, e.g. formal ether and Baermann method.
4. An ELISA test is useful to detect antibodies against excretory—secretory antigen of stongyloides.
5. Other immunological test like immunofluorescence test and radical allergosorbent test (RAST) are promising.

6. An agar plate method that relies on the use of inverted microscope to identify tracks made be motile *Strongyloides stercoralis* larvae. This method is more sensitive than other techniques.

Treatment

Since strongyloidosis is a potentially life-threatening disease so it must be treated properly even if it is asymptomatic. Thiabendazole is drug of choice. It is given as 25 mg/kg body weight twice daily for 2 days. This treatment is extended to 7 days in disseminated stronglyloidiasis. Eosinophilia is a bad prognostic sign.

Prevention Measures

1. Avoid contact with fecally contaminated soil
2. Specific treatment to patients must be given
3. To avoid hyperinfection syndrome, patients must be screened for strongyloidosis, before starting corticosteroids and other immune suppressive therapy.

ENTEROBIUS VERMICULARIS

Synonyms

- Threadworm
- Pinworm
- Seatworm
- Oxyuria

History

- Eggs of thread worm have been found in 10,000 years old coprolith in USA
- Leukart in 1865 described complete life cycle of *Enterobius vermicularis*.

Geographical Distribution

- It has cosmopolitan distribution
- It is more prevalent in temperate and cold climates because of less frequent bathing and less frequent changing of underclothing
- Incidence is higher in developing countries.

Habitat

- Adult worms inhabit in cecum, appendix and ascending colon
- They live in close contact with mucosa.

Morphology

Enterobius vermicularis exists in adult form and larval form.

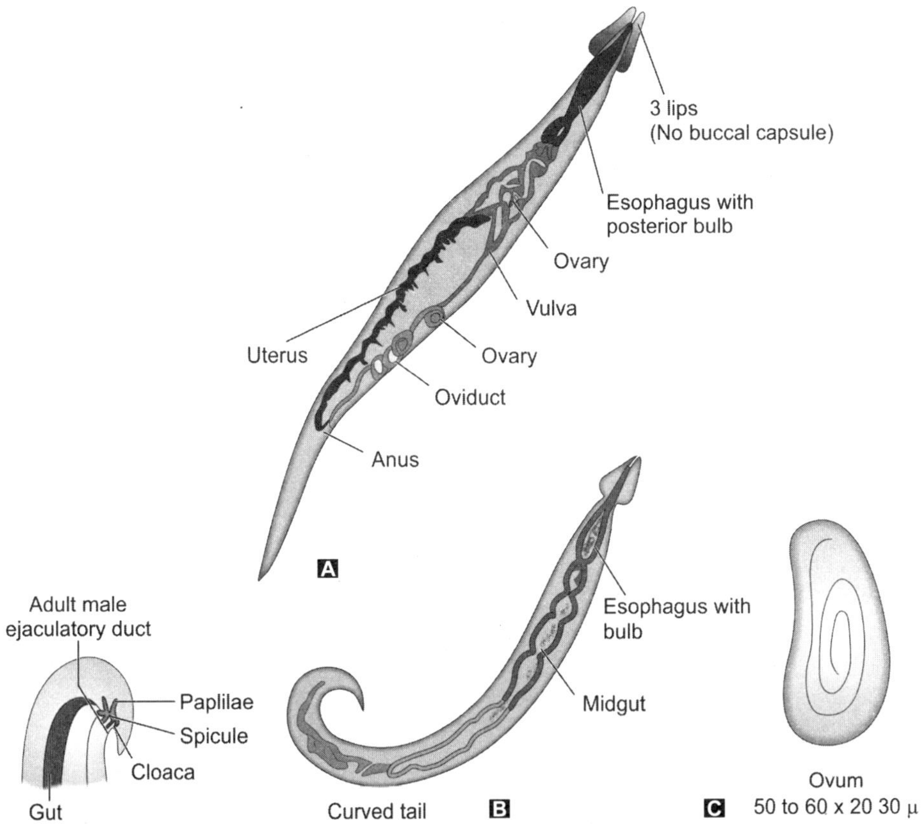

Figs 3.7A to C: Morphology of *Enterobius vermicularis*: (A) Female, (B) Male, (C) Ovum

Adult Worm

- There are wing like expansions at the anterior end of the worm called cervical alae.
- There is characteristic double bulbed esophagus.
- The male worms 2 to 5 mm × 0.1 to 0.2 mm. It has coiled tail with single spicule.
- The female worm is 8 to 13 mm × 0.3 to 0.5 mm with posterior third of body pointed like a pin and is also named pinworm. It is oviparous.
- Male worms live for about 7 weeks while females survive 5–13 weeks.
- Eggs are colorless (non-bile stained) with clear shell, plano-convex in shape and measuring 55 μ × 10 μ. Egg encloses fully formed larva. Eggs float in saturated saline solution.

Life Cycle

- *Enterobius vermicularis* requires one host to complete life cycle and man is the host
- Embryonated egg, (infective form) seek entry to man through feco-oral route
- Eggs hatch in intestine to liberate larvae which develop into mature form in large intestine of the host
- They are differentiated into male and female worms
- The male worm fertilized female worm and dies.

- The gravid female worm migrates out of anus and lay upto 10,000 eggs on perianal area usually at night time
- Larvae within the egg develop fully in 6 hours time. Such mature eggs are infective and may reinfect the same host or reach a new host
- Reinfection in same host (autoinfection) occurs either by hand to mouth route or by a process of retrograde infection. In retrograde infection larvae hatch out perianal region and migrate back through anus upto cecum to further develop there
- Perianal region eggs may contaminate night clothes and bedding. Thus, infection may spread by handling contaminated clothes. Furthers transmission may occur through contaminated hands. Also eggs dispersed around in the environment during bed making may be inhaled. These inhaled eggs stick to mucosa of pharynx and are swallowed. Life cycle is completed in a month time.

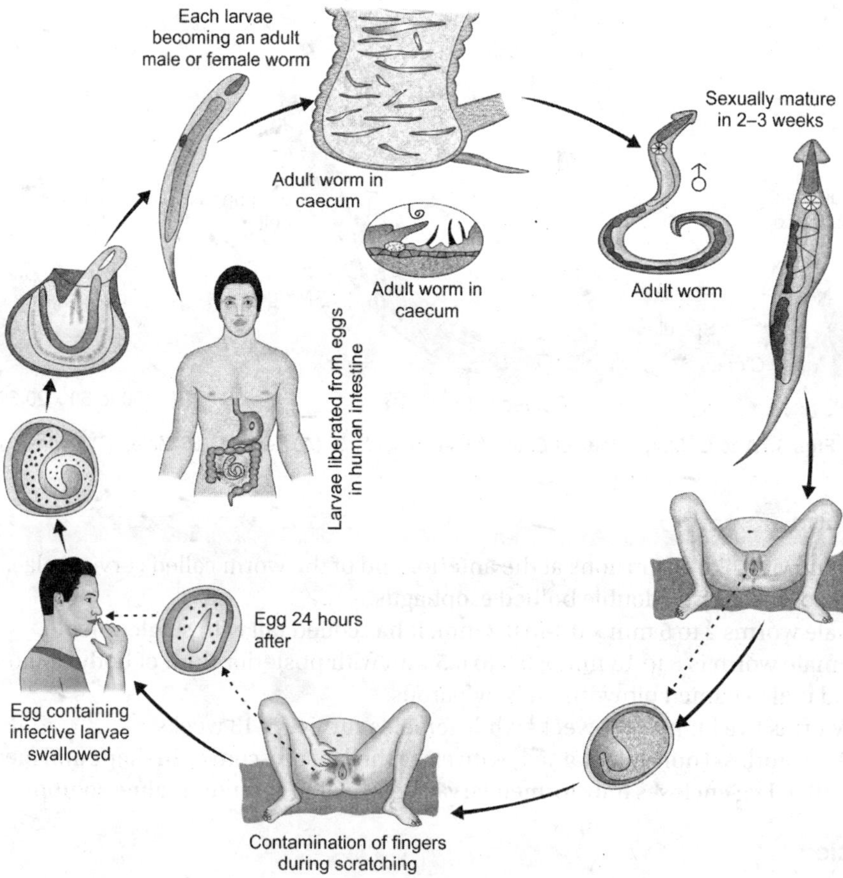

Fig. 3.8: Life cycle of *enterobius vermicularis*

Pathology

It may seek to extraintestinal areas by utilizing small abrasion in the mucosa of gut as it lacks buccal apparatus suited to tissue penetration. It may spread to lungs, liver, spleen, etc. In intestinal enterobiasis there may be ulceration and sumucosal abscesses.

Dead worms and eggs have been identified in granulomata in serveral sites, i.e. vagina, cervix, fallopian tubes, omentum peritoneum, liver, kidneys and lungs.[7]

In extraintestinal areas there may be eosinophilic plus lymphocytic infiltration, ulceration, necrosis and granuloma formation.

Clinical Features

- May be a symptomatic
- Perianal pruritis is characteristic feature of enterobiasis
- Itching is worst at night time
- Excoriation and bacterial super infection may occur
- Nocturnal enuresis may occur
- In females it may cause vulvo-vaginitis, salphingitis and pelvic or peritoneal granulomas
- It may cause appendicitis
- Nail biting.

Laboratory Diagnosis

- Detection of adult worms in perianal region or on the surface of stools is possible. They are also detected in the appendix during appendectomy
- Demonstration of eggs from perianal and perennial region may be done especially at night by scrapping with National Institute of Health (NIH) swab. NIH swab is made up of glass rod at one end of which a piece of transparent cellophane is wrapped and held in place with rubber band. This glass rod fixed in a rubber stopper is kept in a test tube. The cellophane part is rolled over perineal and perianal area and kept back in a test tube and transported to the laboratory for further processing. In the laboratory cellophane is detached and spread over glass slide and examined microscopically. This may be repeated on 3 successive days.
- Eggs may also be recovered form fingernails and washing from undergarments
- As compared to other intestinal nematodes this worm is not associated with pronounced eosinophilia or with elevated IgE.[8]

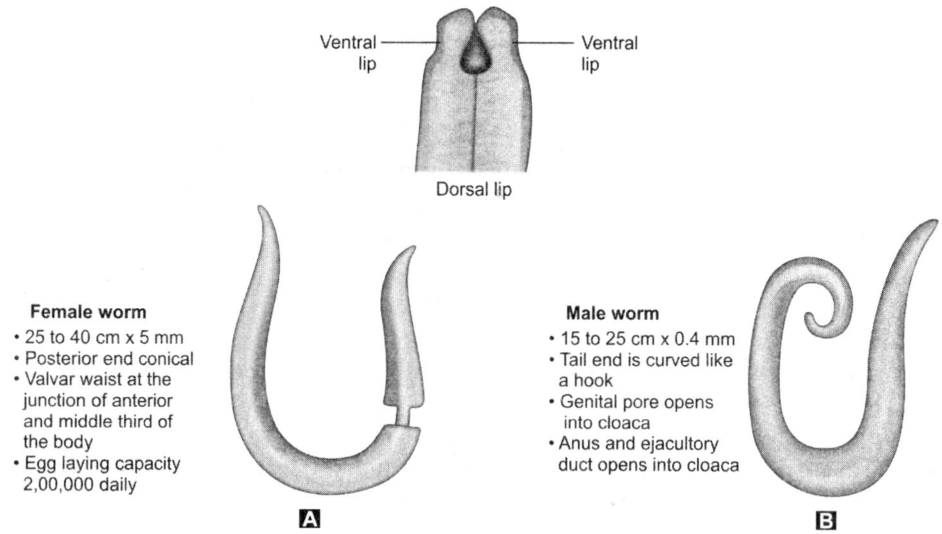

Figs 3.9A and B: Adult worms of *Ascaris lumbricoides*: (A) Female, (B) Male

Treatment

- Pyrantel pamoate may be given in single dose 11 mg/kg of body weight
- Mebendazole in single 100 mg dose is given
- Albendazole as single dose of 400 mg is administered
- Piperzine in a dose of 65 mg per kg body weight is given for 7 days
- All members of the family should be given treatment and may be repeated after 2 weeks.

Preventive Measures

- Finger nails should be kept short
- Frequent hand washing after defecation and before meals
- Adequate personal hygiene must be maintained
- Proper treatment of infected person in particular including other family members
- Fingers should not be put in mouth
- Frequent changing and washing of bed linen and night cloths
- Preferably wearing of gloves by infected persons.

ASCARIS LUMBRICOIDES

Synonym

Roundworm.

History

Discovered by Linnaeus in 1758.

Geographical Distribution

- It is cosmopolitan with worldwide distribution
- Especially prevalent in tropical countries, i.e. India and China
- It affect around 25% world's population
- Highest prevalence is in malnourished persons residing in developing countries.

Habitat

The adult worm resides in small intestine especially in jejunam of humans.

Morphology

- *Ascaris lumbricoides* exist in two forms adult and larvae
- Adult roundworm are the largest intestinal nematodes
- Worm expelled freshly are pinkish and cylindrical
- The anterior end when examined with lens, shows a mouth surrounded by 3 finely toothed lips
- The life span of worm is 1–2 years
- The worm are not attached with intestinal mucosa rather they maintain themselves in the intestine with the help of their muscle tone

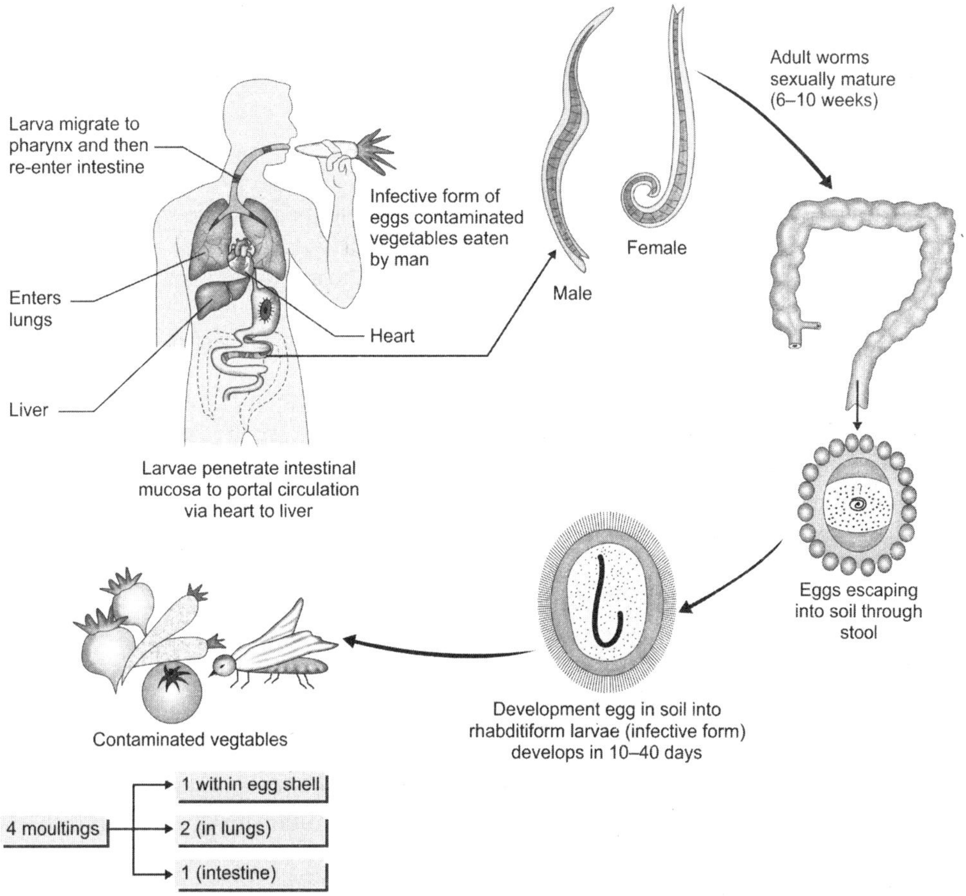

Fig. 3.10: Life cycle of *Ascaris lumbricoides*

- Male adult worm measure 15-30 cm in length and 2-4 mm thick with their posterior end curved and it carries two copulatory spicules
- Female adult worm is 20-40 cm long and 3-6 mm thick with its conical and straight posterior end
- The vulva lies at the junction of anterior and middle third of the body. This part of the worm is narrow and called vulvar waist.
- *Ascaris lumbricoides* is oviparous. Female adult produces upto 2 lakhs egg in a day which are discharged through stools
- The eggs may be unfertilized or fertilized
- Fertilized eggs are 60 μ × 40 μ in size and yellow brown (bile stained) enclosed in egg shell is an unsegmented ovum. There are clear crescentic space at both poles. They are surrounded by a thick, transparent shell consisting of a relatively nonpermeable innermost lipoidal vitelline membrane, a thick transparent middle layer and an outermost coarsely mammillated albuminoid layer. Fertilized egg floats in saturated saline solution of common salt.

- Unfertilized eggs are narrower, longer and measure 90 μ × 35 μ. They are brown (bile stained) in color and contain small atrophied ovum. They have thin shell with irregular coating of albumin. They do not float in saturated saline solution. Unfertilized eggs are produced by female worm. It occurs in the absence of male worm.

Life Cycle

- The worm requires only one host, i.e. human to complete the life cycle
- Embryonated fertilized infective eggs on reaching small intestine liberate larvae
- The motile larvae penetrate through intestinal mucosa to arrive portal circulation to reach liver
- After 3–4 days in liver, the larvae reach systemic circulation via hepatic vein, inferior vena cava, right heart and pulmonary artery to reach the lungs
- Here they grow in size and moult twice (5th day and 10th day)
- Larvae now break through capillary wall to reach alveoli
- From alveoli, the larvae migrate to the bronchi, tranchea, larynx and crawl over the epiglottis to the pharynx and swallowed
- Through esophagus and stomach they pass through and finally get localized in the upper part of small intestine
- On 25th and 29th day of infection, the larvae undergo another moulting and get transformed to adult worms
- In 6–12 weeks, they become sexually mature and by 12th week gravid females start laying eggs which are discharged through feces into soil
- The fertilized eggs containing unsegmented ovum have to undergo incubation in soil to attain infectivity
- Rhabiditiform larvae develops from unsegmented ovum and undergo moulting within egg shell in 10–40 days. The optimal temperature and humidity for development of larvae within the egg is 22–30° C and 40% and more respectively
- These egg containing rhabidatiform larva is infective and which may be taken along with edibles by human thus repeating life cycle.

Pathology

- Infarct or gangrene may develop because of intestinal obstruction, volvulus, etc.
- *Ascaris lumbricoides* may occasionally pass through placenta[9]
- At the site of ectopic ascariasis acute inflammation may occur with infiltration of eosinophils mononuclear and histocytes cells
- Granuloma may be formed around ova in tissues
- Adult worm and larvae secrete allergens which in turn produce IgE by host leading to reaction and histamine production.

Clinical Feature

- Adult worms affect the nutritional status of the host resulting to malnutrition, night blindness due deficiency of vitamin A and ultimately leading to retardation of growth
- The presence of adult worm in intestine may cause colicky cramps and loss of appetite. In case of heavy infection, obstruction and intussusception of intestinal tract may occur

- Adult worms may crawl up and through mouth comes out or may enter nasal meatus via nasopharynx and pass out of a naris. From oropharynx worm may enter eustachian tube penetrate to the middle ear and through tympanic membrane to external auditory meatus. If it enters trachea, respiratory obstruction may occur. It may cause appendictis, obstructive jaundice and acute hemorrhagic pancreatitis. Adult worm is capable of perforation of intestinal wall weakened by ulcers and gangrene
- It may cause allergic manifestations like fever, urticaria, angioneurotic edema, wheezing and conjunctivitis by toxic body fluid (ascaron) released by adult worm inside body of host
- Migrating larvae may result to inflammatory and hypersensitivity reactions in the lungs. It may cause, fever, cough, dyspnea, urticarial rash and eosinophilia. The sputum is blood tinged and may contain ascaris larvae and Charcot Leydin crystals. Thus comprising a syndrome called Loeffler's syndrome. Migrating larvae because of allergic inflammatory reaction may involve liver and kidneys
- Humans acquire only partial immunity to reinfection, and animals may be protected using extract of adult or larvae[10]
- Ascariasis is the most common cause of abdominal surgical emergencies in children in South Africa and Rangoon.[11,12]

Laboratory Diagnosis

1. Demonstration of adult worms in stools. Adult worm may pass through anus, nose and sometime through ear too.
2. Larvae of ascaris may be visualized microscopically in sputum in eosinohilic pneumonia.
3. Demonstration of eggs by direct microscopy or concentration methods like salt floatation method. The eggs may be fertilized or unfertilized. In case of only male worms, eggs are not seen in stools.
4. Plain X-ray, barium studies and ultrasound may show worms in intestines and aberrant sites.
5. Sero diagnosis is good method to detect *Ascaris lumbricoides* antibody. Here methods like indirect hemagglutination immunofluorescence antibody tests and ELISA are used. These methods are especially useful to diagnose extraintestinal ascariasis, e.g. Loeffler's syndrome. These tests are useful for serosurveys too. However, their utility is limited because of cross reactions.

Treatment

- Pyrentel pamoate in single dose of 11 mg/kg maximum upto 1 gram
- Mebendazole can be administered in a dose of 100 mg twice daily for 3 days
- Piperazine citrate in a dose of 75 mg per kg body weight daily for 2 days
- Albendazole as a single dose of 400 mg.

Prophylaxis

- Proper disposal of human stools
- Proper treatment of parasitized persons
- Avoidance of eating raw vegetables and salads
- One must take care of personal hygiene

- Community based chemotherapy periodically in heavily infected group that lack sanitary facilities.

ANCYLOSTOMA DUODENALE

Synonyms

Hookworm and the old world hookworm.

History

- *Ancylostoma duodenale* was described first of all by Dubine in 1843 in Italy
- Life cycle of this worm was reported by Loss in 1898 in Egypt.

Habitat

Adult worm lives in small intestine of man especially in jejunum and less oftenly in duodenum.

Geographical Distribution

- It is prevalent in tropic and suptropic countries especially in Asia, Europe and North Africa
- It occurs mostly in cooler and dry regions
- It is prevalent more in North India.

Morphology

It occurs in 2 forms adult and larval. Adult worms live in small intestine especially in jejunum of humans. They are reddish brown when freshly passed, curved with concavity on the dorsal aspect. The anterior end is bent dorsally hence called hookworm. The mouth has 4 pointed teeth 2 pairs of vertical teeth and 2 blunt teeth on dorsal aspect. Life span of adult worm is 6–8 years. Adult male measures 8–11 mm × 0.4 mm. Its posterior end carrries conspicuous umbrella like copulatory bursa having 2 copulatory spicules. The bursa has membranous lobes (2 laternal, 1 dorsal). These lobes are supported by 13 fleshy rays (3 rays in dorsal lobe and lateral lobes carry 5 rays each).

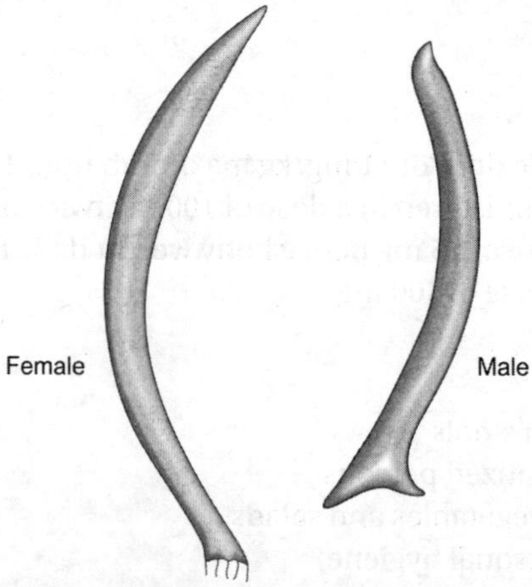

Fig. 3.11: Morphology of *Ancylostoma duodenale*

The adult female measure 10 to 13 mm × 6 mm. Its posterior end is tapering. The vulva opens ventrally at the junction of middle end posterior third of body. It is oviparous and lays 10,000 to 25,000 eggs per day that pass through stools.

Eggs are oval and about 60 μ × 40 μ in size. They are colorless (non-bile stained) with thin hyaline transparent shell. Ovum in the egg is usually segmented with four blastomeres. Eggs float in saturated saline solution. Eggs are not infective as such. They need development in the soil as a result the eggs hatch to produce rhabditiform larvae which grow to filariform larvae (infective form).

Life Cycle

- Life cycle is completed in only one host, i.e. humans.
- Eggs are passed along stools and develop in the soil. As a result rhabiditiform larvae hatch out from egg in about 48 hours.
- Rhabditiform larvae moult twice to develop into filariform larvae which is infective form of larvae.
- The time taken following deposition of eggs in soil to develop into filariform larvae is 8–10 days.
- Filariform larvae penetrate skin (mostly foot) of humans.

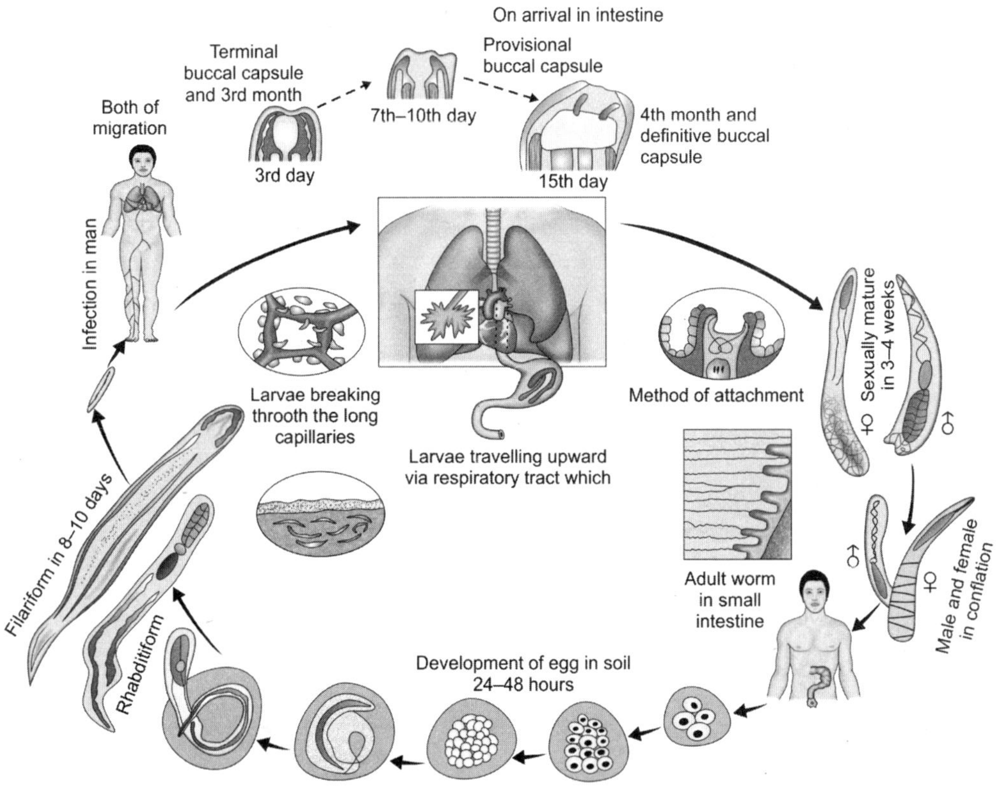

Fig. 3.12: Life cycle of *Ancylostoma duodenale*

- From skin they invade blood stream to reach lungs and from here they penetrate through capillaries to reach alveoli
- From alveoli larvae ascend the bronchial tree, trachea, larynx, pharynx and through epiglottis are swallowed through saliva to stomach and then to jejunum
- In jejunam larvae get attached with mucosa and develop intu adults in 3–4 weeks time. Male fertilizes female and female ultimately liberate eggs which are passed with the stool of the patient into the soil where the eggs develop into infective larvae infecting new host and this cycle repeats. The prepatent period following skin invasion to the appearance of eggs in the stool takes around about 6–8 weeks
- During entire life cycle hookworm moults four times. In soil it moults two time to acquire mouth parts required for penetration of skin, blood vessels and alveoli. In pharynx esophagus of humans, filariform larvae moults once to get a temporary buccal capsule required for tis attachment. The fourth multing takes place to acquire regular buccal cavity.

Pathogenesis

Important pathological features are as under:

- In creeping eruption, there is lymphocyctic and eosinophilic infiltration seen in upper layer of dermis
- The principle histological findings in the lungs include eosinophilic infiltration and edema which are due to allergic reaction
- Intestinal mucosa may show petechial hemorrhages, superficial erosion, congestion and edema. Mucosa and submucosa show infiltration by eosinophils, lymphocytes and plasma cells.

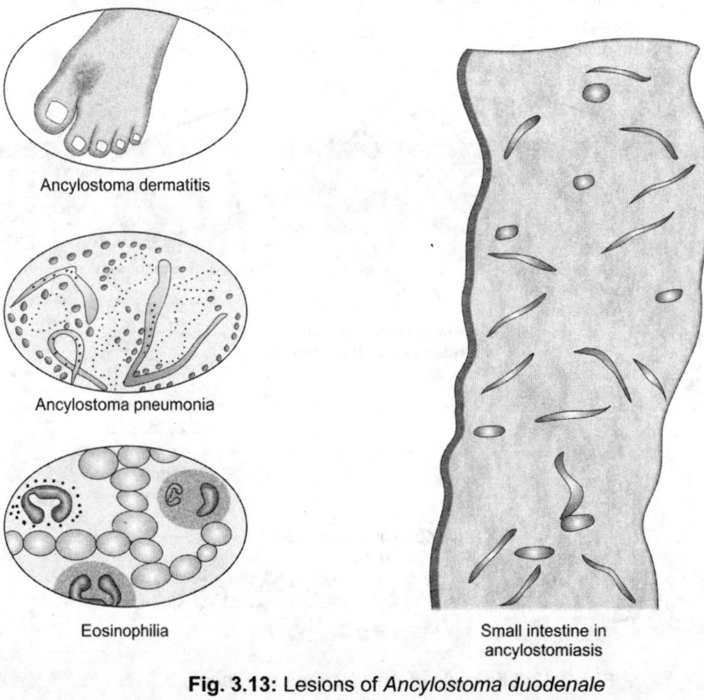

Fig. 3.13: Lesions of *Ancylostoma duodenale*

- Intestinal villi may show blunting, atrophy and fusion due to associated malnutrition
- Histological diagnosis is made only by demonstration of parasite.

Clinical Features

Skin

- Local erythema
- Maculopapular rash
- Intense prutitis.

Lungs

- Cough
- Wheezing and rales
- Wakana disease encountered more in Japan highlighted by pulmonary manifestations and hypereosinophilia.

Gastrointestinal

- Epigastric discomfort
- Nausea associated with vomiting
- Anorexia
- Diarrhea
- Pica
- Hemorrhage.

Miscellaneous

- Iron-deficiency anemia which may be because of:
  - Chronic blood loss from hemorrhages in jejunum because of hookworm
  - Blood sucking by hookworm
  - Suppression of hemopoietic system (bone marrow) usually due to deficient protein consumption
- Dyspnea, edema, fatigue, etc.
- Depletion of iron stores

Laboratory Diagnosis

Direct Methods

- Demonstration of typical eggs in stool by direct microscopy or concentration methods. About 2000 eggs per ml of stools in women and children and 5000 eggs per ml in males is associated with significant anemia
- Adult worms may be visualized in stools
- Eggs and adult worms may also be demonstrated from aspiration of duodenum obtainable by Ryle's tube
- Stool may be cultured using Harua Mori filter paper strip or charcoal culture method.

Indirect Methods

- In peripheral blood film one may find microcytic hypochromic anemia and eosinophilia
- Stool examination may reveal occult blood and Charcot Leyden crystals

Treatment

- Anemia if present must be treated along with anthelminthic drugs
- Mebendazole 100 mg twice daily for 3 days may be used
- Pyrantel pamoate in the dose of 11 mg/kg body weight is effective
- Albendazole 400 mg in single dose may be used as treatment
- Thiabendazole or bephenium hydroxynaphthoate or tetrachloroethylene are the other alternative drugs.

Prevention and Control

- Proper sewage disposal to prevent fecal soil contact
- Prevention of human contact by using barriers like gloves, shoes, etc.
- Edible should be properly cleaned and must be eaten after washing hands
- Treatment of persons infected with hookworm.

Necator Americanus

Features

- The adult *Necator americanus* is smaller and slenderer as compared to *Ancylostoma duodenale*
- The anterior end bends in the opposite direction to the body curvature
- The buccal capsule bears four chitinous plates (2 ventral and 2 dorsal)
- Adult male worm is 7 to 9 mm × 0.3 mm with its copulatory bursa long and wide
- Copulatory bursa has 14 rays of which dorsal ray is split from base. Both of the copulatory spicules are fused at the ends
- Female adult measures 9 to 11 mm × 0.4mm. The vulva is placed in the middle of the body
- Adult worm sucks 0.03 ml of blood in day
- Otherwise pathogenicity, clinical features life cycle, laboratory diagnosis, treatment, prevention and control methods are almost same as those of *Ancylostoma duodenale*.

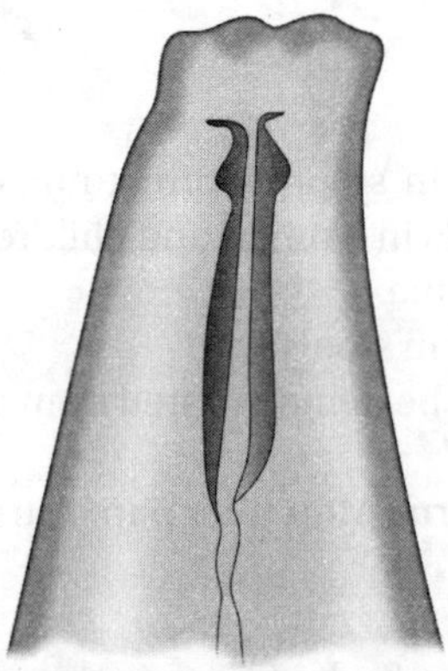

Fig. 3.14: Morphology of *Necator americanus*

ANCYLOSTOMA BRAZILIENSE

Features

- It is a hookworm of dogs and cats in India, Brazil and Malaysia
- Adult worms are much smaller to that of *Ancylostoma duodenale*
- Buccal capsule has small orifice
- Dental plate bears one pair of large teeth
- Male bursa is small in size and supported by short lateral rays
- The eggs resemble with those of *Ancylostoma duodenale*
- Its filariform larvae cannot penetrate underneath the level of stratum germinativium and hence unable to have access to blood vessels. It finds ways to small intestine and result in cutaneous larva migrans.

CLONORCHIS SINENSIS

Synonyms

- Opisthorchis sinensis
- Chinese liver fluke
- Diatoma sinensis.

History

- *Clonorchis sinensis* was first described in 1875 by Mc Connel in the bile passages of Chinese carpenter in Calcutta (India)
- Detailed life cycle were worked out in 1927 by Faust and Khaw.

Geographical Distribution

- It is mainly confined to Orient, from Vietnam to Japan
- The endemic areas like Japan, South Korea, China, etc.
- In other areas of the world, imported cases occur from Asia.

Habitat

- The adult worm lives attached within the small intrahepatic bile ducts
- In heavy infection adult worms may be found in extrahepatic bile ducts, pancreatic ducts and gallbladder.

Morphology

Adult worm

- It is narrow, oblong, flat worm with pointed anterior and rounded posterior end
- It measures 10–25 mm in length by 3–5 mm in broad
- The oral sucker is slightly larger than ventral sucker which is present at the junction of anterior and middle third of the body
- The blind intestinal ceca are simple and extend to the caudal end
- It has large, deeply lobulated branched testes
- Testes are situated one behind the other
- Worm can live in biliary tract upto 50 years.

Eggs

- They are broadly ovoid
- They have moderately thick, light yellowish brown shell (bile skinned)
- They bear distinct convex operculum on their shoulders
- At posterior end there is small knob
- They measure 28 to 35 μ × 12 to 19 μ
- They contain ciliated embryo i.e. miracidium when discharged inside the bile duct
- They do not float in saturated saline solution of common salt
- The hatching occur only after ingestion by molluscan hosts.

Infective Form

- Metacercae in a flesh of fresh water fish is the infective form of parasite.

Life Cycle

- Life cycle of *Chlonorchis sinensis* requires, Three hosts, one definite and two intermediate hosts
- Definite hosts may be human, dog, cat or pig
- Firsts intermediate host is snail (bulimus)
- Second intermediate host may be fish belonging to cyprinidae family or cray fish (*Caridina, Paloemonetes sinensis*)
- Fully embryonated eggs containing miracidium are discharged with stools of definite host into water
- These eggs are taken up by suitable species of snail (*Bulimus* or *Alocinma*) and miracidium hatches out from egg.

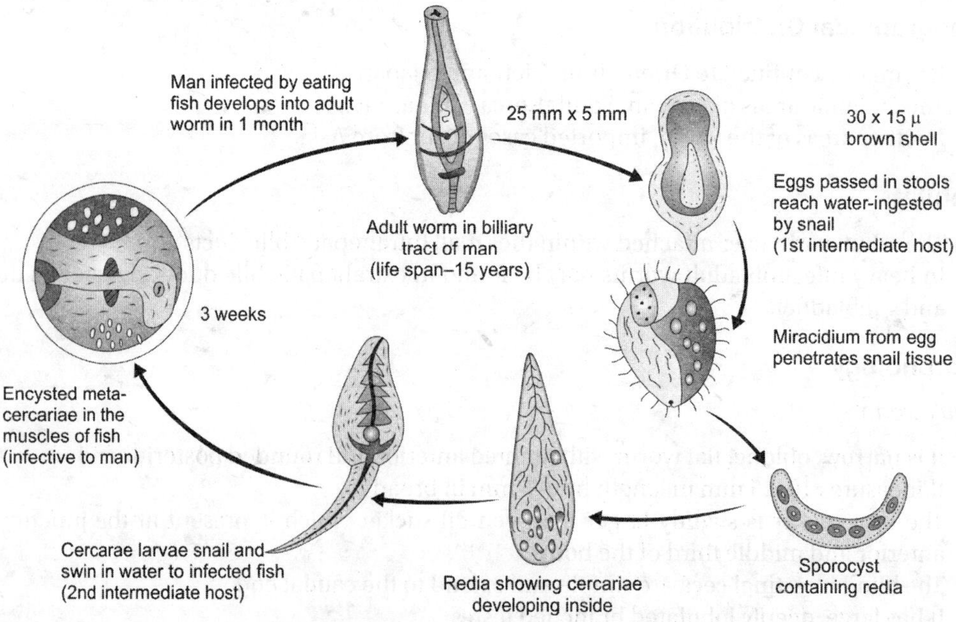

Fig. 3.15: Life cycle of *Clonorchis sinensis*

- Within the snail first generation sporocyst and the second generation rediae develop which grow to cercariae
- After coming out of snail, cercariae swim in water and on coming in contact with fresh water fish (cyprinidae or cray fish), cercarae get attached to fish, discard their tail to penetrate under scales to encyst in skin or in flesh
- Ingestion of infected fish by human makes the encysted cercariae (metacercariae) to excyst in duodenum. They enter the common bile duct through the ampulla of vater, where they mature in a month time
- The mature worm results in proliferation of biliary epithelium, increased muern secretion, etc.
- Recurrent attacks may cause biliary obstruction
- Adult worms may infect pancreatic ducts, periductal fibrosis causing acute pancreatitis The eggs are discharged through stool and thus life cycle is repeated.

Pathogenesis

- Thickening and localized dilation of bile ducts is noticed in heavy infection. There may be hyperplasia of small mucinous glands of the duct mucosa
- The adenomatous changes may persist for many years
- These changes because of infections may result into adenocarcinoma of bile duct, hepatocellular carcinoma and cholangiocarcinoma.

Clinical Features

- Light infections are asymptomatic
- Worm load of 500 to 1000 flukes often give rise to clinical signs and symptoms
- During migration of larvae person may develop fever, tender hepatomegaly, mild jaundice, and eosinophilia.

Laboratory Diagnosis

- Demonstration of eggs by microscopic examination of stools or aspirated bile by duodenal aspiration
- Differential leukocyte count with 10–40% of eosinophilia
- Serological diagnosis is done by ELISA, complement fixation test and indirect hemagglutination test
- Skin test using extracts of adult *Clonorchis sinensis.*

Treatment

- Praziquantel is the drug of choice. It is administered in the dose of 40 mg/kg body weight or 25 mg/kg body weight for 3 doses space 8 hours apart is recommended treatment
- Albendazole is equally good
- Bithionol in the dose of 30–50 mg/kg body weight may be given orally on alternative days for 2–3 weeks.

Prevention and Control

- Raw or uncooked fish should not to be eaten
- Freezing at -10°C for 5 days or salting in 10% solution can kill metacercarae

- Sanitation improvement and health education is a must
- Proper disposal of humans, cats and dogs stools.

FASCIOLOPSIS BUSKI

Synonyms

- Distomat buski
- Giant intestinal fluke.

History

- Buskin in 1843 described *Fasciolopsis* buski first of all. Adult worm was detected in the duodenum of dead East Indian sailor that time who died in London.

Geographical Distribution

- China
- Thailand
- Myanmar
- Malaysia
- In India, it is prevalent in:
  - Assam
  - West Bengal.

Habitat

- Adults are seen in small intestine especially duodenum of humans and pigs. Pig is a normal host which acts as a reservoir of infection in humans.

Morphology

Adult worm

- Largest trematode parasitizing in humans
- It is elongated ovoid with anterior end narrower than posterior end
- It is 20–75 mm in length, 8–20 mm in breadth and 0.5–3 mm in thickness
- Cephalic cone is absent
- Oral sucker measures 0.5 mm and lies closer to acetabulum which is 2–3 mm in diameter
- Two intestinal ceca are without any branch
- Life span of worm is around 6 months
- They live in small intestine.

Eggs

- It is pale yellow brown, large and oval
- It measures 140 μ × 85 μ
- It contains unsegmented ovum surrounded by many yolk granules
- Egg granules in yolk cells are uniformally distributed and not concentrated around nucleus as seen in *Fasciola hepatica*

- The shell is clear, thick and possesses a small operculum which is difficult to visualize
- It does not float in saturated saline solution
- It can develop only in water
- The eggs of *Fasciolopsis buski* are difficult to differentiate from Fasciola hepatica
- Each worm lays about 25000 eggs per day.

Infective Forms

- Metacercariae are encysted on aquatic vegetation. This metacercariae infected vegetation may be ingested by humans.

Life Cycle

- The adult worm remains attached to the mucosa of duodenum and Jejunum of human and pigs
- The immature eggs are discharged in the stools and they reach fresh water
- The miracidia develop inside the eggs in about 3–7 weeks in summer
- Micacidia come out of eggs, swim around in water and ultimately succeed in coming in contact with snail (*Segmentina* and *Hippeutis*) the first intermediate host. They penetrate soft tissue of snail and in few weeks time develop into sporocyst first and second generation radiae. Ultimately cercariae are produced

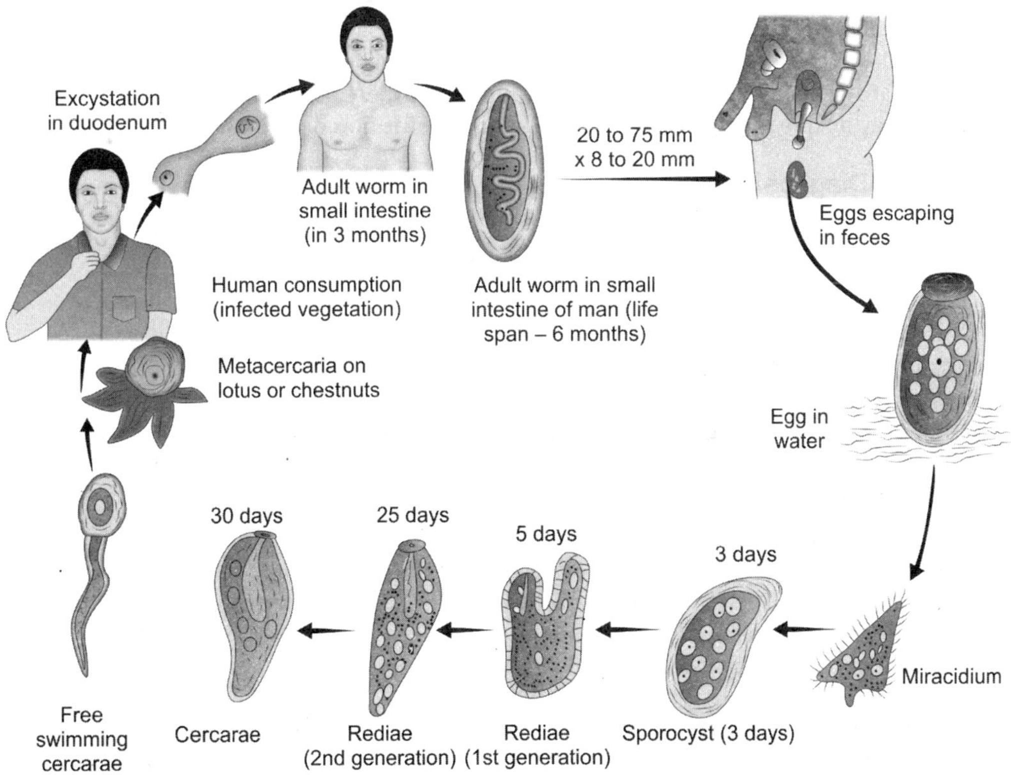

Fig. 3.16: Life cycle of *Fasciolopsis buski*

- Cercariae come out of snail and encyst on seed pods of water caltrop, the bulb of the water chestnut, roots of lotus, water bamboo and other aquatic vegetation (second intermediate host)
- Humans get infection by peeling off skin of these infested plants. They do so by keeping these plants between teeth and lips before swallowing the raw nuts
- In the process metacercariae excyst in the duodenum and become adhered to the intestinal wall and grow into adult worms in about 3 months
- Eggs are liberated which are discharged through stool and the cycle is repeated.

Pathology

- In mild cases lesions are seen only in duodenum and Jejunum
- In sever cases ileum, colon and stomach may be involved
- In mild cases mucosa is edematous and congested. In severe cases hemorrhages and superficial ulcers are also observed
- Additionally in severe cases there may be cystic dilatation, crypt abscess and lymphoid hyperplasia.

Clinical Features

- Most infected persons may be asymptomatic
- Clinical feature are mainly due to mechanical injury, obstruction, intoxication and allergic manifestation because of metabolic byproducts of the parasite
- Patient may have abdominal pain, diarrhea alternating with constipation, low grade fever, stunted growth and generalized edema. Additionally there may be facial edema and ascites
- Death may be due to intestinal obstruction or malnutrition or both.

Laboratory Diagnosis

- Detection of operculated eggs in stools
- Adult worm can be recovered and identified after purgative and anthelminthics.

Treatment

- Prazinquntel may be administered as a single dose of 15 mg/kg body weight at bed time. The success rate is 100%
- Other drugs like niclosamide or hexylresorcinol may be used.

Prevention and Control

- Adequate washing of water vegetables with hot water
- Storage of feces with lime may destroy eggs in night soil
- Eggs, miracidia and cercaria in contaminated water may be destroyed by using 100 ppm of quick lime or 20 ppm copper sulfate
- Destruction of snails by using 20 ppm of copper sulfate in ponds.

DIPHYLLOBOTHRIUM LATUM

Synonyms

- Fish tapeworm

- Brood tape worm
- Tenia lata
- Bothriocephalus latus
- Dibothriocephalus latus.

History

- It was identified first of all by Dunus in 1592 from Europe
- It was differentiated from Tenia by Plater in 1602
- In 1758 Linaeus named this parasite Tenia lata
- In 1910 Luhe described it as *Diphyllobothrium latum*.

Geographical Distribution

- Northern Italy
- Switzerland
- Germany
- North America
- Japan
- Eastern Canada.

Habitat

The adult worm is located in lower jejunum or upper ileum with scolex embedded in mucosa.

Morphology

They are found in adult form, eggs form and larval form.

Adult Worm

- When freshly expelled from human intestine it is yellowish gray or ivory in color
- It measure 3–10 meters or more in length with about 3000 proglottids
- It is longest tapeworm found in man
- It has scolex, neck and strobilla
- Scolex is spoon, shaped and measures 2 to 3 mm in length and 1 mm in breadth
- Scolex bears two slot like grooves on dorsal and ventral surfaces respectively. However there are no restellum or hooklets
- Neck is situated immediately behind scolex. It is thin, unsegmented and several times the length of the head
- Strobilla bears 3000 or more proglottides (segments) which may be immature, mature and gravid segments. The mature segment is 10 to 20 mm × 2 to 4 mm and filled with male and female reproductive organs. A coiled uterus is lying centrally within each segment. Eggs are discharged through uterine pore of each proglottid
- Single worm may discharge around one million eggs daily. The terminal segments are shrunked and empty. Later the segments get dried up and they break off from body in chains and passed out in stools.

Eggs

- They are yellow-brown in color (bile stained)
- They are oval, elliptical and measure 70 μ × 45 μ and possess thin and smooth shell
- They have ungenmented ovum containing plenty of yolk granules
- They bear unconspicous operculum at one end with a small knob at other end
- They do not float in saturated saline solution of common salt
- The eggs as such are not infective to man.

Larval Form

- The eggs during development pass through first stage, second stage and third stage larva
- First stage larva is coracidium and develops from egg in water
- The preferred second intermediate hosts are temperate fresh water fish especially pike, perch and hurbot[13]
- Second stage larva is percercoid and develop from coracidium inside copepods
- The third stage larva is procercoid which grows from procercoid in fresh water fish.

Life Cycle

- This parasite completes its life cycle in one definitive host (man, dogs, cats, foxes, bears, pigs, etc.) and two intermediate hosts. Small copepods and Cyclops fishes are first intermediate host and fresh water fishes are second intermediate host
- Adult worms live in small instestine (ileum jejunum) of humans and other definitive host. They liberate operculated eggs which are passed out with stools and they find way into water. The eggs develop to form spherical ciliated embryos with three pairs of hooklets each. It takes 1–2 weeks times. This hexacanth embryo or oncosphere develops into coracidium
- Coracidium swims around in water and is eaten by copepods. In order to continue the development coracidium must be ingested by copepods within 12 hours
- In the intestine of copepod, ciliated embryophore is shed. Now oncosphere penetrate the intestine of copepod and enters body cavity. Here it is transformed into procercoid form in 2–3 weeks time. It measures 0.5 mm in length
- Now copoepods with infective procercoid larvae are eaten by second intermediate host, i.e. fresh water fish. The procercoid penetrate the intestine of fish and reach between muscle fibers and grow to plerocercoid larvae measuring 10 to 20 mm × 2 to 3 mm
- Plerocercoid larvae is neither encysted nor encapsulated. It is well developed with partly invaginated scolex
- This small infected fish may be eaten by larger fish. Plerocercoids succeed in penetrating the intestine of second host where they survive without development
- Humans are infected on consumption of raw or undercooked or lightly salted meat from infected fresh water fish
- In the intestine of humans plerocercoid larva develops into adult worms attaining sexual maturity in 5–6 weeks
- Eggs are liberated which move out along with stools into water and cycle is repeated.

Pathogenicity

- *Diphyllobothrium latum* grows and liberate metabolic wastes into human intestinal lumen. Its pathogenic effect is directly related to mass of worm, type of byproducts absorbed into hosts tissue, hosts susceptibility to these foreign products, etc.

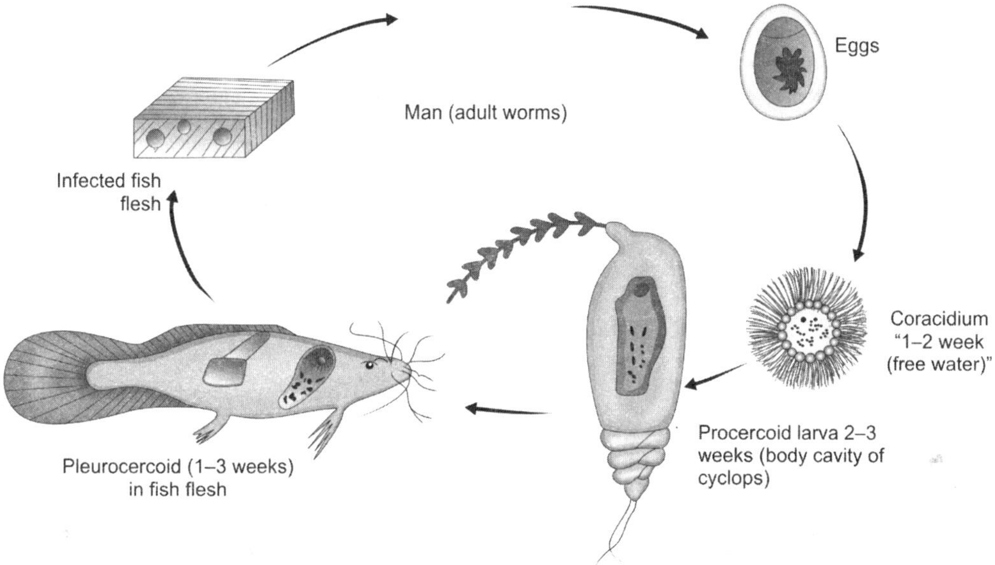

Fig. 3.17: Life cycle of *Diphyllobothrium latum*

- Because of attachement of worm to wall of ileum there is imbalance between intrinsic and extrinsic factors of Castle resulting into pernicious type of anemia. Consumption of large amount of vitamin B_{12} by this parasite, deprive the host of essential nutritional components causing pernicious anemia
- Leukocytosis and eosinophilia is significant changes encountered in this infection.

Clinical Features

- In most of the cases infection is asymptomatic
- In some cases abdominal pain and mild diarrhea may occur
- In 2% cases megablastic anemia may occur because of parasite prevents vitamin B_{12} absorption by combining with intrinsic factor and blocking vitamin B_{12}
- Some patients suffers from sensation of hunger, singing in the ear, craving for salt, fatigue, weakness and numbness of extremities
- Occasionally vomiting of worms and intestinal obstruction may be observed in few patients.

Laboratory Diagnosis

- Demonstration of segments of the worm by undertaking microscopic examination of feces. However in reference laboratories electrophoretic methods like isoenzyme characterization are helpful in the identification of parasite
- Demonstration of eggs of *Diphyllobothrium latum* is possible. The eggs remain viable upto 1 year in refrigerated stool samples. The samples may also be preserved in 10% formalin. Since large number of eggs are discharge through stool so direct wet mount is usually positive. In negative cases a concentration method is also beneficial
- Serological techniques like ELISA, latex agglutination can be used with encouraging results.

Treatment

- Three drugs effective to treat this parasite include niclosamide, praziquantel and bithionol
- Since cure is not 100% hence examination of stool samples for eggs or scolex may be repeated 3 weeks after treatment
- Other drugs effective are quinacrine hydrochloride, parmomycun, etc.
- Pernicious anemia may require administration of folic acid 20–30 mg daily for 7-10 days.

Prevention and Control

- Thorough cooking of suspected fresh water fish is important
- Efficient disposal of sewage
- Prevention of pollution of water
- In endemic areas of infection cats, dogs should not be fed with raw or undercooked fish
- Carriers should be taken care of properly
- Health education.

HYMENOLEPIS NANA

Synonyms

- Dwarf tapeworm.

History

- First of all reported in 1857 by Bilharz
- Its life cycle was elucidated during 1887 to 1892 by Grassi and Rovelli.

Geographical Distribution

- It is cosmopolitan in distribution
- It is predominant in warm climate
- It is particularly common in India, Europe and USA.

Habitat

The adult worm lives in the lumen of upper three quarters of ileum of human.

Morphology

Adult worm

- It is small and thread like
- It measures 1 to 4 cm × 1 mm
- Adult worms are usually found in large number 1000 to 8000 in intestine
- Its life span is about 2 weeks
- It comprises of scolex neck and strobilli
- Scolex is globular and bear four cup shaped suckers and a refractile rostellum armed with single raw of 20–30 hooklets
- Neck is long, slender and lies posterior to the scolex

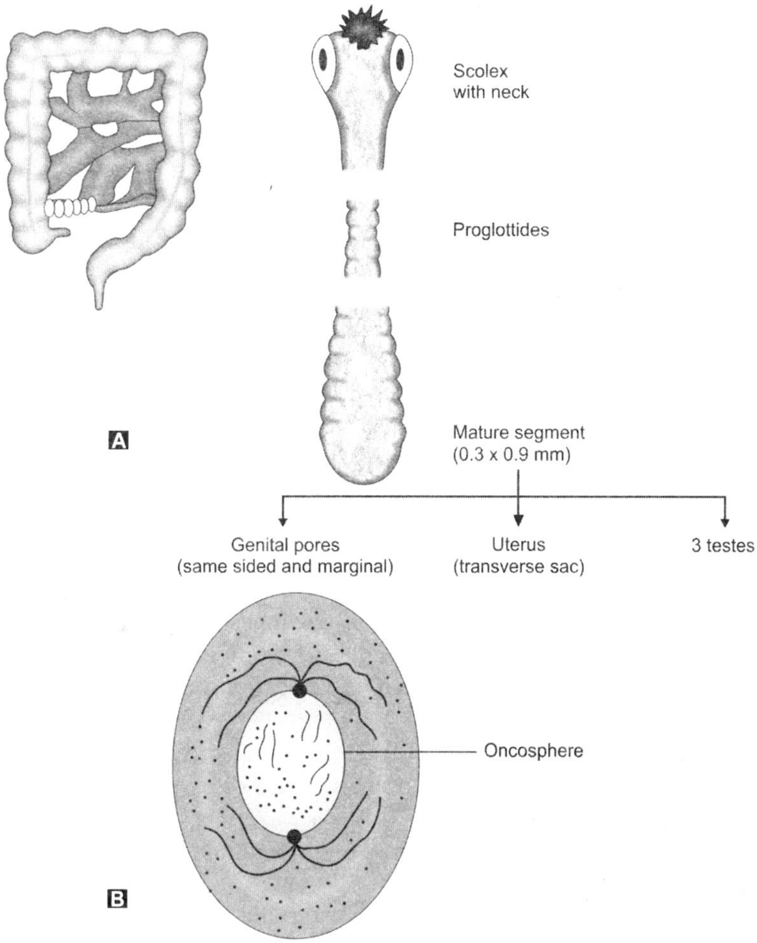

Figs 3.18A and B: Morphology of *Hymenolepis nana* (A) Adult worms, (B) Eggs

- Strobilli consists of 200 proglottides. A mature proglottid measures 0.15 to 0.3 mm × 0.8 to 1 mm. Genital pores lie marginally and on the same side. The gravid uterus forms a sac like structure with lobuated wall filled with 80 to 200 eggs
- Testes are three in number and are round shaped.

Eggs

- They are colorless and oval
- It measures 45 μ × 35 μ
- The egg has thin colorless outer membrane and an inner embryophore enclosing hexacanth embryo
- The space between two membranes contain yok granules and 4 to 8 thread like structure called polar filaments which arise from two knobs of embryophore
- Oncosphere contains three pairs of hooklets
- Eggs float in saturated salt solution
- It is non-bile stained.

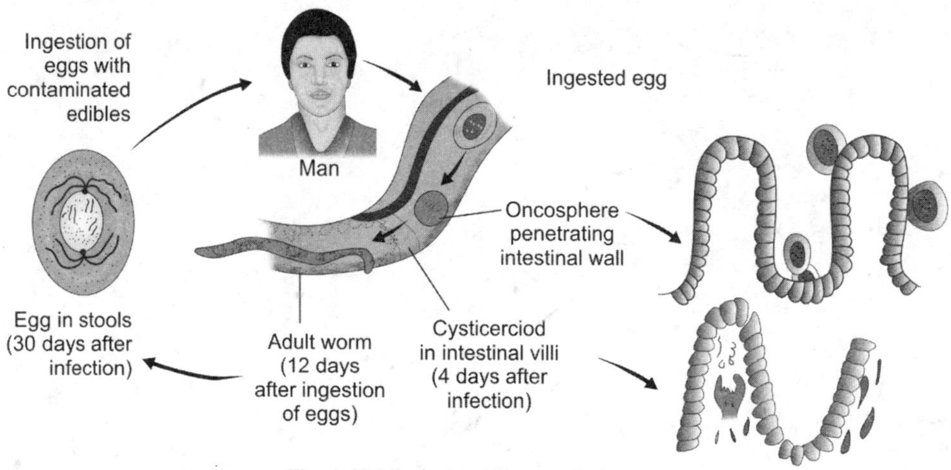

Fig. 3.19: Life cycle of *Hymenolepis nana*

Life Cycle

- It takes place only in one host and no intermediate host is required
- Fully embryonated eggs freshly passed in stools are ingested by humans
- The eggs are hatched in the stomach or small intestine and free oncosphere penetrate into villi of the anterior part of small intestine and transform into young cercocysts or cysticercoids
- These larvae now migrate into lumen of small intestine and get attached by the scolices to other villi further down in small intestine. In coarse of 2 weeks' time they develop into mature worms
- Strobilization (production of new segments) is quite rapid and in 30 days after ingestion the adult worms start liberating eggs
- Some of the eggs are passed along with stools restart life cycle in same host, i.e. human
- *Hymenolepis nana* is the only tapeworm typically utilizing no intermediate host
- This parasite is one of the exception to general rule that helminths do not multiply inside the body of definite host. This is direct life cycle
- In indirect life cycle rat flea (Xenopsylla cheopis) and beetle acts as intermediate host and transmit the infection from mice to humans.

Pathogenicity

- The villi of ileum are damaged by cysticerci of *Hymenolepis nana*
- Likewise adult worm is also capable of producing mechanical damage to mucosa
- There may be protein losses from the small intestine. Protein absorption and digestion will be disturbed
- Increased activity of intestinal enterokinase and phospholipase is observed
- The peroxidation of erythrocytic membrane is increased in proportion to the duration and severity of infection[14]
- Serveral reports have shown association with retardation of growth in hymenlepsiasis.[15]

Clinical Features

- Patients carrying few worms in intestine are asymptomatic
- In heavy infection patients may develop abdominal discomfort, diarrhea and anorexia
- Autoinfection usually leads to hyperinfection. It happens mostly in immunocompromised patients.

Laboratory Diagnosis

- Demonstration of eggs which are characteristic and are identified by microscopic examination of stools (direct preparation, salt floatation or formalin ether concentration techniques)
- Repeated examination is invariably needed because eggs liberation in stool may be irregular
- An enzyme linked immunosorbent assay (ELISA) has been developed with sensitivity of about 80%.[16]

Treatment

- Drug of choice is praziquantel which is given in proper doses. It is quite effective. Single dose of 25 mg/kg body weight is sufficient
- Alternatively niclosamide may be administered. It is given in dose of 2 g daily for 5–7 days. In heavy infection second coarse may be given after 10 days.
- Family members eight instructional mates should be treated simultaneously. It would minimize the risk of infection from out side.

Prevention and Control

- Improved sanitation is the main factor toward prevention
- Change of behavior especially in children is emphatically underlined. To clean perioneal region after defecation with hands dirt (dust) must be discouraged
- Mass chemotherapy does play an important role to prevent and control this parasitic infection
- Rat and mice control programme might reduce the incidence of infection.

TAENIA SAGINATA

Synonyms

- The beef tapeworm
- The unarmed tape worm
- Asian tenae
- Tenae african
- Tenie hylnchus saginatya
- Tenae confuse
- Tenae hominis.

History

- It is known since ancient times
- Goez differentiated it from pork tapeworm in 1782
- Leukart in 1861 demonstrated first of all that cattle are intermediate host of this parasite.

Geographical Distribution

- *Taenia saginata* has worldwide distribution and is found wherever beef is consumed
- Area of high prevalence includes:
  - Iran
  - Taiwan
  - Philippines
  - USA
  - Germany
  - UK
  - India (muslim dominating areas).

Habitat

The adult worm lives in the upper part of jejunum with scolex embedded in the mucosa of intestine.

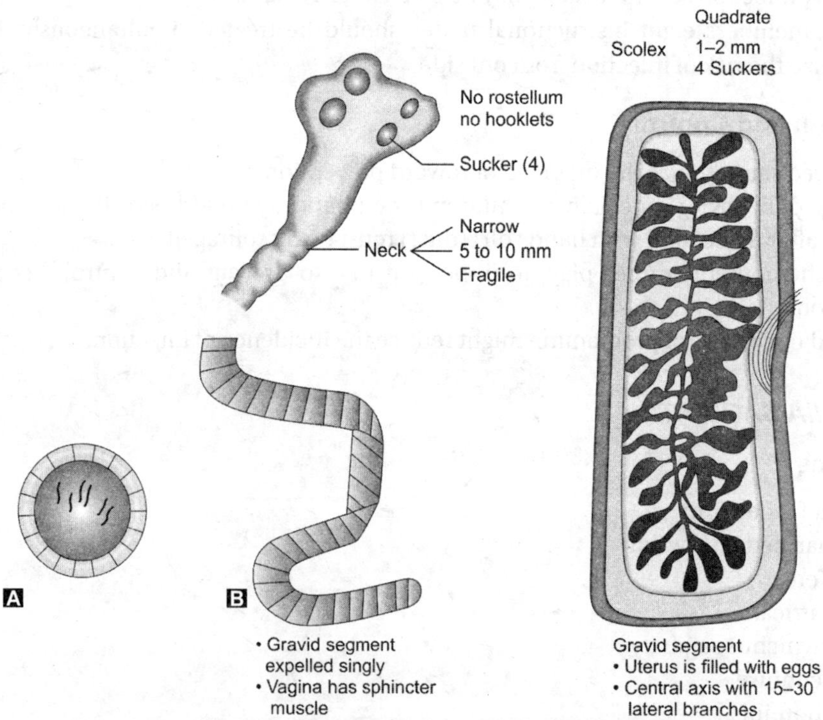

Figs 3.20A and B: Morphology of *Taenia saginata,* (A) Eggs, (B) Adult worms

Morphology

Adult Worm

- It is a whitish and semitransparent worm
- It is 5–10 meters long and sometimes it may be 24 meters long
- It is largest helminth infecting man
- The scolex is 1–2 mm in diameter, quadrate in shape, each angle has four circular sucker (pigmented) with which it is attached to intestine. No hooklets are present on head hence called unarmed worm
- The neck is long, fragile and narrower than the head, 0.5 mm in width
- The proglottides or segment are 1000 to 2000 in number comprising of immature, mature and gravid arranged from front backwards
- The gravid segments are 3 to 4 times longer than they are broad (2 cm × 0.5 cm)
- The common genital pore is placed marginally at the hind end of each segment alternating irregularly between right and left margins
- From the longitudinal uterus 15 to 30 lateral branches emerge on each side
- The number of lobes of ovary is two and number of testes is 800 to 1200
- There is a muscular sphincter attached to vagina
- The gravid proglottid is detached singly and passes actively through anal opening, ovipositing on perianal skin
- Each gravid segment may contain 80,000 to 1,03,000 eggs
- Longevity of worm is over 30 years.

Eggs

- It is spherical brown in color (bile stained) measuring 31μ × 43 μ
- It is surrounded by embryophore which is brown colored, thick walled. That is radially striated
- Outside this may be present thin transparent shell which represent remnant yolk mass
- Inside embryophore lies hexacanth embryo (oncosphere) with three pairs of hooklets
- It does not float in saturated saline solution
- These eggs are infective only to cattle.

Life Cycle

- Cows or buffaloes at the time of grazing in the field ingest gravid segments passed out in the stools of definitive host on the ground
- After ingestion, they come to duodenum where embryophore of eggs rupture discharging onchospheres
- With the help of the hooklets oncosphere penetrate the wall of intestine and find their way into portal vessels or mesenteric lymphatics.
- They reach general circulation through liver, right side of heart, lungs and finally to left side of heart
- From general circulation they are filtered out in striated muscles and in 10–12 weeks they grow into bladder worm called cysticercus bovis
- The mature cysticerci are ovoid in outline milky white, opalescent measuring 7.5–10 mm and invaginated

- These can live in flesh of cattle for almost 8 months and develop further only when eaten by humans
- Humans get infection by consuming raw or undercooked beef containing encysted larvae (cysticercus bovis)
- On reaching small intestine the larvae hatch out the scolices exvaginate and get attached with mucosal surface by suckers. They develop into adult forms, get sexually mature in 2–3 months and lay eggs
- The eggs are passed out through stools along with gravid segments. They reach the ground and taken by cows or buffaloes during grazing in the field. Hence cycle is repeated.

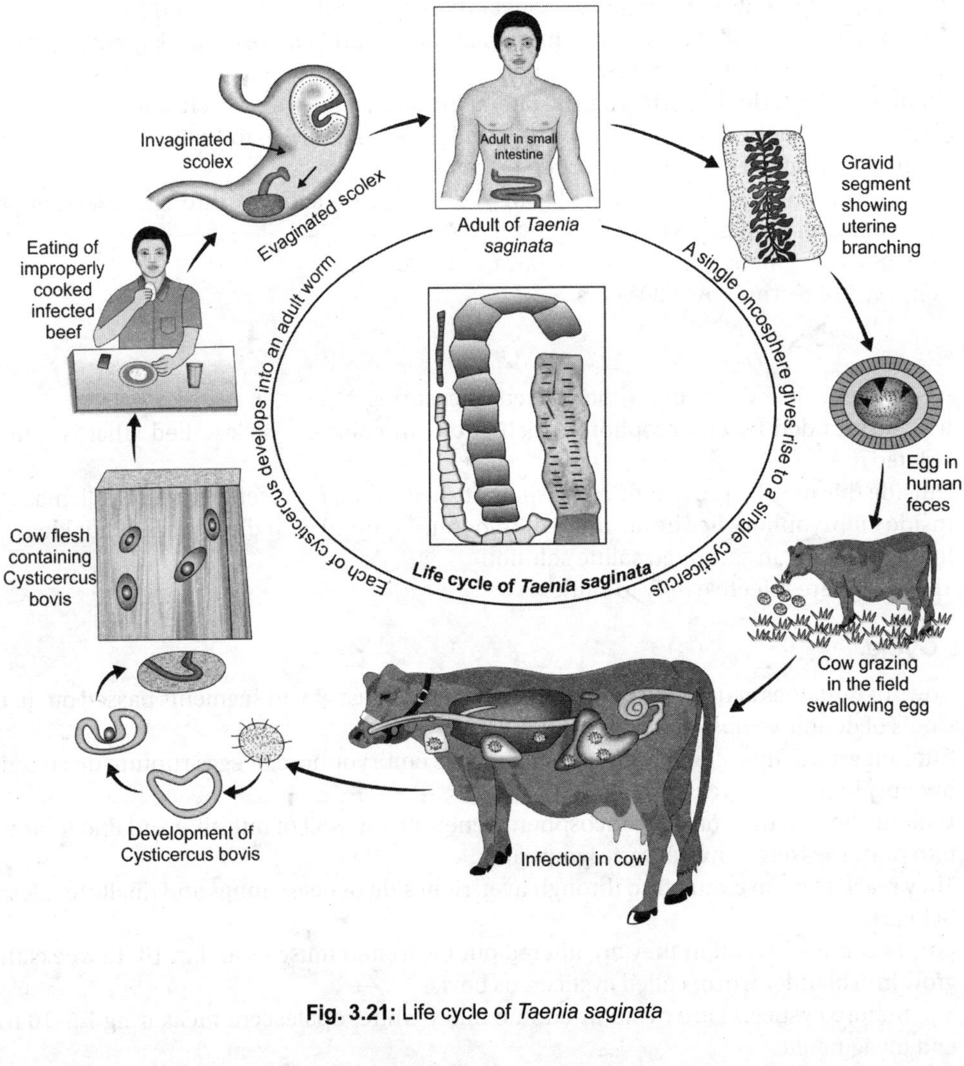

Fig. 3.21: Life cycle of *Taenia saginata*

Pathogenicity

- It causes changes in secretion of gastrointestinal tract
- Gastric secretion is reduced in 70% of infected patients
- Irritation because of worm may cause flatulence, cramps and diarrhea
- The mature tapeworm remains attached to the upper Jejunum with posterior part of the body down to ileum. However, tapeworm is mobile in intestinal lumen.[17]

Clinical Picture

- Usually asymptomatic
- Expulsion of proglottides through anus
- Abdominal discomfort hunger pain, chronic indigestion, diarrhea alternating with constipation, etc. may be present
- Anorexia
- Neural disorder
- Intestinal obstruction associated with appendicitis may occur.

Laboratory Diagnosis

- Demonstration of proglottides or eggs is possible. They are seen in stools of patients or undergarments
- A perianal NIH swab is useful to demonstrate eggs
- Serodiagnosis is useful tool in diagnosing *Taenia saginata* infection. Tests which are in use are indirect hemagglutination, indirect fluorescent antibody and ELISA
- Soluble tenia antigen can be detected in stools but present method tend to be cross reactive.[18]

Treatment

- Niclosamide 2 g as a single dose in the morning on an empty stomach is administered. Tablet must be chewed first before swallowing. The worm may come out within few hours otherwise purgative must be administered. This drug is effective n 90% of patients. It is very safe drug and can be given safely in pregnancy
- Praziquantel is effective in 90% patients. It is given in doses of 5 to 10 mg/kg body weight as single dose after a light breakfast.
- Treatment given is considered successful if no proglottid come out within 4 months after taking treatment.

Prevention and Control

- Raw or undercooked beef must not be consumed. The cysticercae are killed at 48°C
- Meat should be inspected thoroughly at slaughter house
- Proper sanitation, sewage disposal and hygiene in cattle form should be maintained
- Early detection and treatment helps to control infection
- Prophylactic treatment at interval of 3 months to all persons in feedlot is helpful to prevent and control infection
- Lime nitrogen (artificial fertilizer) may shorten the survival of eggs to a considerable extent.

TAENIA SOLIUM

Synonyms

- Tenia cucurbitina
- Pork tapeworm
- Armed tapeworm.

History

- Linnaeus in 1758 discovered this parasite
- Leuckart in 1856 described the life cycle of *Taenia solium* and reported that cysticercus cellulosae present in the muscles of pig was infact infective to man.

Geographical Distribution

- It is prevalent worldwide
- It is common in pork eating population being nil in Muslims and Jews.

Habitat

The adult worm is found in the small intestine of humans.

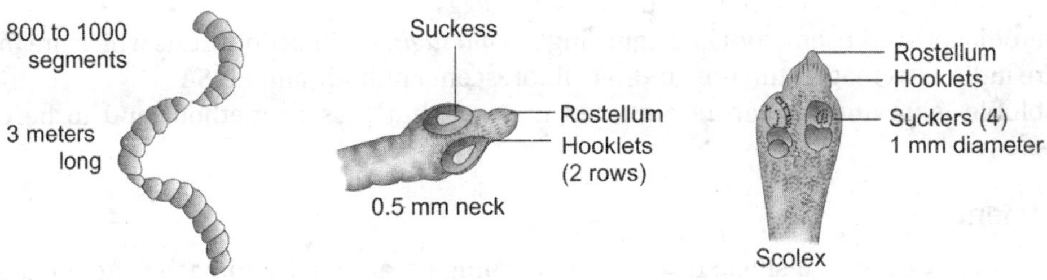

Fig. 3.22: Adult worms of *Taenia solium*

Morphology

Adult worm

- It measures 2-3 meters in length
- Scolex is pin head size, globular in outline and has four suckers. The head bears rostellum armed with double raw of large and small hooklets
- Proglottides are less than 1000 in number. A gravid segment is longer than broader while immediate proglottides are broader than longer. The genital pore may be present laterally at the middle of a each segment alternating between right and left side.
- The testes consists of 150-200 follicles. The ovary lies in the posterior third of each proglottid and consist of two large symmetrical lobes and an accessary lobe. The gravid segments get separated from strobila. They are passed passively in the stools.

Larval Form

- The larval form is called cysticercus cellulosae and occurs in humans
- It is small, avoid, milky white bladder measuring 1 mm × 8 to 10 mm
- It contains fluid rich in fluid and salts.

- The larva lies parallel to muscle fibers showing a small white spot representing the future head invaginated into bladder
- The pork containing cysticerci is reffered to as measly pork.

Eggs

- Eggs resemble structurally with eggs of *Taenia saginata*
- Eggs are liberated through ruptured wall or disintegrated gravid proglottide in stools
- Eggs remain viable for many weeks outside the host. They are infective to pig as well as humans.

Life Cycle

- In *Taenia solium* two hosts are needed to complete life cycle. Humans and pigs are two hosts
- The infective form of parasite for humans is cysticercus cellulosae
- Humans are infected by taking raw or improperly cooked pork containing cysticercus cellulosae. Digestion of the pork in the intestine liberates scolex

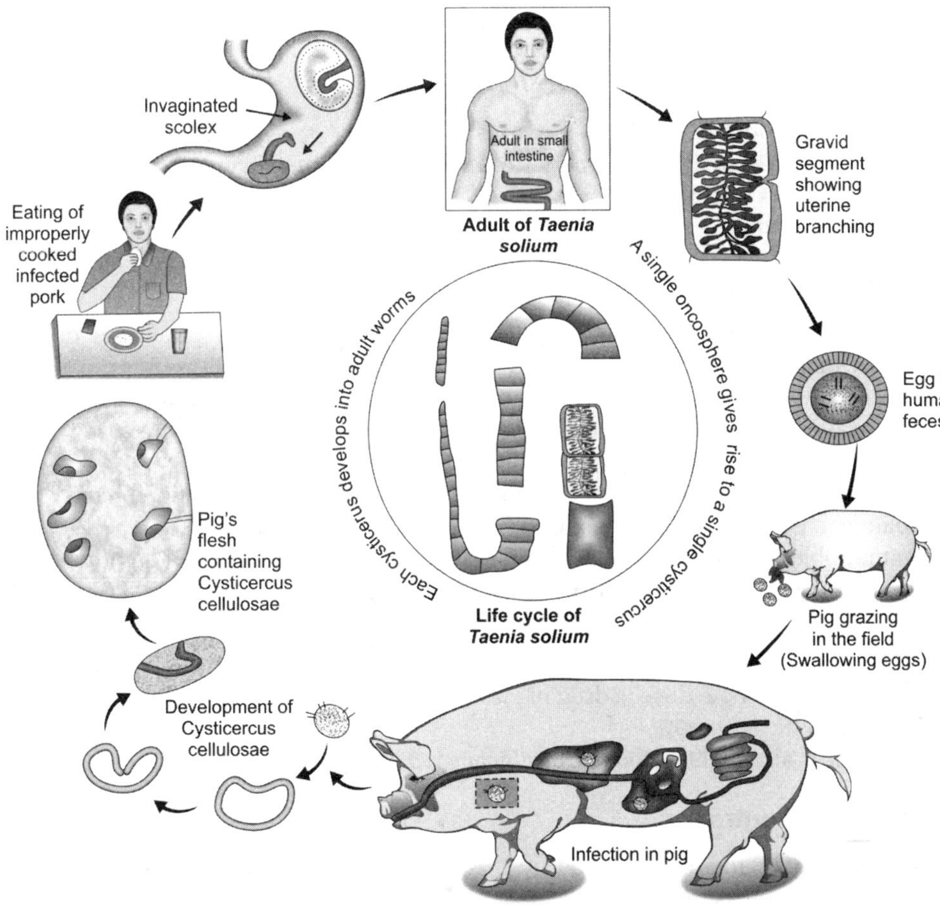

Fig. 3.23: Life cycle of *Taenia solium*

- The scolex evaginates and get adhered to the intestinal mucosa with the help of suckers and hooks
- Progressive strobilization results to growth of adult worm which get matured in 2–3 months after infection
- Gravid segments develop after completion of fertilization in mature segments. Now gravid segments or eggs may pass through stools
- The eggs may survive for several weeks in soil
- The life cycle starts in the pig by ingesting these viable eggs
- Hexacanth embryo is liberated in the intestine of pig, penetrates the gut wall with the help of hooklets to reach the blood stream
- From blood stream embryos are primarily filtered in the muscles of neck, shoulder, leg and tongue
- The embryos on settling in muscles transform into bladder like structure called cysticercus cellulosae and it takes 60–70 days
- When pork infected with cyticerucus cellulosae is eaten raw or undercooked by humans and life cycle repeats.
- Ingestion of edibles contaminated water containing egg can also initiate life cycle in humans.

Clinical Picture

- It may be asymptomatic in most of the cases in humans
- However there may be diarrhea, abdominal pain, loss of appetite, etc.
- Main problem is experienced because of cysticercus cellulosae mainly manifest as subcutaneous nodules.

Laboratory Diagnosis

- Demonstration of proglottides or eggs is quite informative. The proglottides of *Taenia solium* are identified by examining scolex which is armed with rostellum. It is most reliable feature to identify *Taenia solium*. Finding of eggs only suggest and not confirm the diagnosis
- Demonstration of gravid proglottide and count of lateral branches of uterus (5–10) suggest specific pre-treatment diagnosis
- Serodiagnosis by indirect hemagglutination, ELISA and IFA using *Taenia solium* coproantigen is reasonably promising
- An immunoblot assay that may be 95% sensitive and 100% specific for serodiagnosis of *Taenia solium* easily differentiable from *Taenia saginata*.[19]

Treatment

- Praziquantel in a single dose is drug of choice. It is administered in dose of 10–15 mg/kg body weight. Efficacy is 90%
- Niclosamide is also highly effective. Its efficacy is 90%.

Prevention and Control

- Personal hygiene is to be maintained
- General sanitary measures
- Avoidance of consumption of raw or undercooked pork and vegetable irrigated by water

- Rigid quality inspection of pork in slaughter house
- Avoidance of fecal contamination either from self or other infected with adult worms
- Infection with adult worm can be checked if we heat the pork meat at 49 ° C to 53° C for minimum 30 minutes or freezing it at –5 °C for 3 days which kill the larvae.

CYSTICERCUS CELLULOSAE

Synonym

Taenia solium cysticercus.

Geographical Distribution

- It is found in all regions where *Taenia solium* is prevalent
- They are found as under:
  - South and Central America
  - South and East Africa
  - Russia
  - India.

Morphology

- Fully developed cysticercus cellulosae is 10 mm × 5 mm in dimension, opalescent with ellipsoidal body
- It bears opaque invaginated scolex with four suckers and hooks
- It encloses fluid filled bladder
- Cysticercus cellulosae lies parallel to muscle fibers
- The developing time is 7–9 weeks
- Cysticercus cellulosae occur in cattle. They develop in humans as under:
  - By ingesting eggs with contaminated water and food (raw vegetables irrigated with sewage water)
  - Humans having adult worms may autoinfect themselves by virtue of their unhygienic habits or by reverse peristaltic movement of intestine resulting to push back gravid segments into the stomach which means swallowing of numerous eggs.

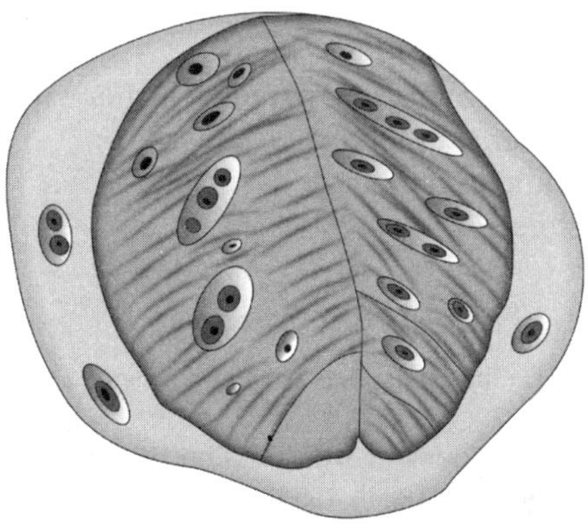

Fig. 3.24: Cysticercus cellulosae

Pathogenicity

- Cysticercus cellulosae may develop in any organ and the effects so produced depend on the location of cysticercae
- They oftenly involve subcutaneous tissues and muscles ultimately forming nodules
- They may develop in brain resulting to epileptic seizures
- They may involve anterior and vitreous chambers of the eye.

Clinical Picture

- Subcutaneous nodules
- Jacksonian type of epilepsy
- Hydrocephalus
- Encephalitis
- Blurred vision or blindness
- Diplopia
- Aphasia and amnesia.

Laboratory Diagnosis

- Biopsy is helpful in diagnosing this disease. Histopathological study is done of suspicious involved tissue
- Serological tests are useful, e.g. indirect hemagglutination, indirect fluorescent antibody, and ELISA
- Radiological tests like X-ray of skull and soft tissue may show calcified cysticerci
- CAT scanning or MRI can detect cysticerci in central nervous system. Ocular cysts can be spotted by ophthalmoscopy
- Fine needle aspiration cytology is useful
- Immunoblot and immunoelectrotransfer blot using blood for antibody detection in neurocysticercosis are beneficial.

Treatment

- Surgical removal is recommended if possible
- Two drugs, i.e. praziquantel and albendazole are effective.

Prevention and Control

- Hygienic measures like good sanitary and personal hygiene must be followed carefully
- Early treatment of patient of *Taenia solium*
- Adequate cooking of pork and vegetables
- Vaccination of pigs if feasible.

REFERENCES

1. Capo V and Despommier. DD clinical aspects of infection with *Trichinella* spp. Clin Microbiol Rev. 1996:47–54.
2. Campbell, WC. Epidemiology Modes of transmission. In Compbell WC (Ed.), *Trichinella* and *trichinosis*, New York: Plenum Press, 1983b:425-44.
3. Bundy DAP and Cooper ES. *Trichuris* and *Trichuriasis* in humans 1989;28:107–73.

4. Holland CV. Neglected infections trichuriasis and strongyloidiasis. In Stephenson LS (Ed). Impact of Helminth Infections on Human Nutrition. London: Taylor and Francis 1987b:161-201.
5. Berk SL, Verghese A, et al. Clinical and epidemiologic features of strongyloidiasis. Arch Intern Med, 1987;147:1257-61.
6. Iwamoto T, Kotoh M, et al. Larva currens: The usefulness of the agar plate method. Dermatology, 1998;196:343-5.
7. Cook GC. Entrobius vermicularis infection. In Farthing MIG, Keusch GT, Wakelin D (Eds). London: Chapman and Hall, 1995:213-23.
8. Jarret EEE and Karr JW. Thread worms and IgE in allergic asthma. Clin. Allergy 3;203-7.
9. Da Costa Macedo, Rey LM. *Ascaris lumbricoides* in neonate evidence of congenital transmission of intestinal nematodes. Rev Inst Med Trop Sao Paulo, 1990;32:351-4.
10. Williams JF and Souls by EJL, Antigenic analysis of the development stage of Ascaris suum. Exp. Parasitol. 1970; 27:150-62.
11. F Loue JH. Abdominal complications of *Ascaris lumbricoides* infection in children. Br J Surg. 1966;53:510-21.
12. Thein - Hlaing *Ascaris lumbricoides* infections in Burma. In: Crompton DWT, Neisheim MC and Pawlowski ZS (Eds). Ascarisis and its Public Health significance, London, Taylorand Francfis, 1985:83-112.
13. Muller R. Worms and Disease William Heinmann Med. Book Ltd. London. 1975;161.
14. Kartasheva LD. The functional activity of gastrointestinal tract and intensity of peroxidation of erythrocyte lipids in hymenolepsiasis (In: Russia). Med. Parazytol (Mask), 1980; 49:32-37.
15. Khalil HM, el Shimi S, Sarwat MA, Fawzy AF, el Sorougy AO. Recent study of Hymentotepis nana infection in Egyptian Children J. Egypt. Soc Parasitol 1991;21:293-300.
16. Castillo RH, Grados P, Carcamo C, et al. Effect of treatment on serum antibody to Hymenolepis naan detected by enzyme linked immunosorbent assay. J Clin Microbiol. 1991;29:413-14.
17. Prevat R, Hornbostel H and Dorken H. Lokalisationsstudien Bei Tenia Saginata. Klin Wochenschr. 1952;30:78-80.
18. Allen JC, Avila G, Garria-Noval J, Flisser and Craig PS. Immunodiganosis of teniasis by coprantigen detection. Parasitol 1990;101:473-77.
19. Wilkins PP, Allan JC, et al. Development of serological assay to detect Tenia solum teniasis Am. J. Trop Med Hyg. 1999;60:1999-2004.

Tissue Helminths

4

PARAGONIMUS WESTERMANI

Synonyms

- Oriental lung fluke
- Pulmonary distomiasis.

History

Paragonimus westermani was first discovered in the lungs of Bengal tigers by Kerberi in 1878. Later on Ringer et al reported the worm in human autopsy and eggs were found in sputum. Recently over 9 species are reported of this parasite.[1]

Geographical Distribution

- Japan
- Korea
- Manchuria
- China
- South East Asia
- Papua
- New guinea
- Solomons
- Samoa
- In India it is predominant in West Bengal, Tamil Nadu and area around Mumbai.

Habitat

Adult flukes are found in the cystic cavities in the lungs usually in pairs.

Morphology

It occurs as an adult form, eggs form and infective form

Adult Worm

- It is thick flesh, oval shaped, reddish brown in color which is covered with scale like spines
- Its anterior end is relatively broader than the posterior end
- It is 16 mm long, 8 mm wide and 5 mm in thickness
- Ventral sucker lies toward the middle of body
- Similarly oral suckers are situated on the anterior end

- This fluke has a large excretory bladder which extend from posterior extremity to the level of pharynx in the anterior area
- Two blind intestinal caeca are unbranched and may go upto caudal region
- Adult worm can live upto 20–30 years.

Eggs

- Eggs are golden brown, thick shelled oval provided with flattended operculum
- It measure 88–100 μ × 50 μ to 60 μ
- They are unembryonated when laid. It means it contains unsegmented ovum surrounded by yolk cells.

Infective Form

Metacercariae encysted in the flesh of crustaceans, i.e. crayfish, crab, etc.

Life Cycle

- Life cycle is completed in three hosts, one definitive host and two intermediate hosts
- Man, wolf, fox, tiger, leopard, dog, monkey are definitive hosts
- Freshwater snail (semisulcospira and brotia) is first intermediate host
- A freshwater crayfish or a crab (crustacean) is second intermediate host
- Adult fluke lay eggs in cystic cavities of the lungs.
- The eggs may be voided in the sputum or come out via stool from swallowed sputum and reach water
- In the contaminated water, ciliated miracidia hatch after 16 days to 7 weeks
- Now it enters fresh water snail where these miracidia develop into sporocysts, followed by two generations of rediae and finally short tailed cercariae. Time taken for these stages is around 3 months
- The cercariae emerge out of the snails and swim freely in water. They can survive for only 24–48 hours. It order to maintain cycle, they must attack second intermediate host (crabs or crayfish)
- Cercariae penetrate freshwater crustaceans and encyst in the gill, muscles, legs and viscera as metacercariae (250–500μ). Carbs may be infected be ingesting the cercariae in water or by eating infected snail. It requires 6–8 week's time to transform into infective form capable of infecting definitive hosts.
- On consumption of crab or crayfish humans get infection
- Metacercariae reach stomach and hatch in duodenum
- The young worms penetrate wall of small intestine travel across the abdominal mesenteries thus entering abdominal wall in 6 hours
- Burrowing through diaphragm the young flukes enter pleural cavity in 6–10 days
- They now enter the bronchioles of the lung in 15–20 days and form cystic cavities
- They grow and attain maturity and begin to lay eggs in 5–6 weeks of infection
- Eggs are expelled in sputum or may be dislodged by coughing, swallowed excreted in stool and the cycle is repeated
- Paragonimus is a hermophrodite but two worms are necessary for fertilization to occur. A fluke can lay 11000 to 10,4000 eggs per day.

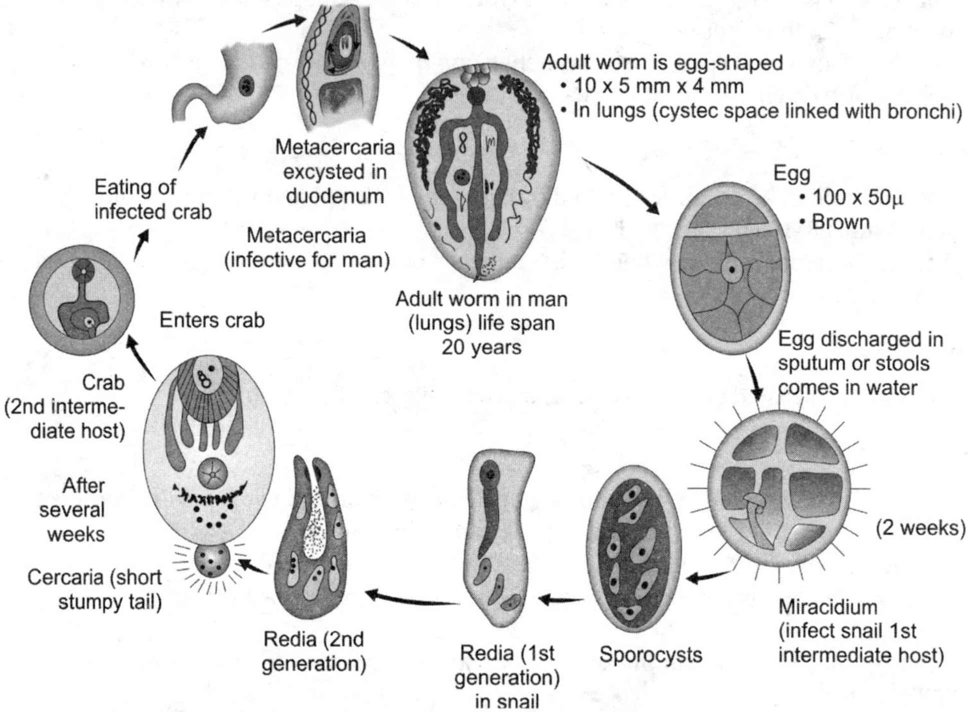

Fig. 4.1: Life cycle of *Paragonimus westermani*

Pathology

- An eosinophilic granuloma may be formed around worm which ultimately is transformed into fibrous cyst
- The pulmonary lesions may be of 1 cm in diameter and freely communicate with bronchioles
- Small fibrous nodules around deposited eggs are found
- Calcification may occur presenting radiological finding resembling tuberculosis.

Clinical Features

- Incubation period is 5–6 months because of migration of worm in lungs. There may be fever, chills, pain and cough. In case of established parasite in lungs there may be malaise, sweating, cough, chest pain, eosinophilia, pleurisy with hemoptysis, pleural effusion, pneumothorax, clubbing, etc.
- Central nervous system may be involved 10 months after pulmonary involvement. Patients develop headache, vomiting, seizures and visual disturbance.
- Hemoptysis caused by *Paragonimus westermani* requires differentiation from that of more prevalent tuberculosis in co-endemic area.[2]
- Bloody diarrhea and abscess in liver and spleen may develop
- In skin lesions patient may develop subcutaneous eosinophilia nodules.

Laboratory Diagnosis

Paragonimiasis must be kept in mind in persons who consume raw or under cooked cray fish and their clinical features hints toward this parasite. Following tests are helpful in establishing diagnosis:

- Peripheral blood and absolute eosinophilic count reveals eosinophilia.
- Demonstration of characteristic yellowish brown operculated eggs in the sputum aspirated pleural effusion or stool. Sputum may be blood tinged having rusty brown flukes.
- Serological tests like ELISA is useful and quite sensitive. The complement fixation tests using veronal buffered saline extract of adult *Paragonimus westermani* antigen correlates reasonably with active infection. Likewise other tests like gel diffusion, immunoelectrophoresis, etc. are also useful.
- Skin test using extract of *Paragonimus westermani* as an antigen is also beneficial.
- Biopsy may be helpful in detecting parasite fragment and sometimes even eggs.
- Radiological diagnosis can be useful in case patchy foci of fibrotic change with characteristic ring shadow.

Treatment

- Praziquantel 25 mg/kg body weight thrice daily for 3 days is quite effective regime.
- Bithiomol may be administered on alternated days for 10–15 days in divided doses of 30–40 mg/kg body weight. The symptoms of disease disappear rapidly. However superinfection should be treated if occurs.
- Another drug niclosamide in single dose of 2 mg/kg body weight is effective. Cure rate is 100%.

Prevention and Control

- Sanitation improvement and health education may be useful to interrupt transmission from sputum and stools. Further education may prevent persons to eat raw, undercooked or smoked crab or crayfish
- Proper treatment of patients with appropriate anthelminthic drugs is undertaken. Thus, transmission of infection is ceased to great extent
- Destruction of molluscan host using molluscicides.

DRACUNCULUS MEDINENSIS

Synonyms

- Guinea worm
- Median worm
- Dragon worm
- Serpent worm.

History

- This worm is refered as fiery serpent in bible
- The worm was detected in 16th century from African country Guinea Bisai hence the name guinea worm.

Geographical Distribution

- Middle East
- Africa
- Pakistan (Eradicated)
- Eradicated from India.

Habitat

Adult female worm are found in subcutaneous tissues of legs, arms and back.

Morphology

Adult Worm

They have rounded head terminating in a thickened chitinous shield containing triangular mouth and papillae.

Adult Male

- It is rarely visualized
- It measure 1.2 to 2.9 cm × 0.4 mm
- Posterior of male worm is coiled on itself once or more times
- Male fertilizes female worm and dies.

Adult Female

- It is a slender and long worm
- It measure 50 to 80 cm × 1 to 2 mm
- It resembles a piece of long twisted thread
- The body is cylindrical, smooth milky white in color,
- Anterior end is blunty rounded. Posterior extremely is tapering and is bent to form a hook
- It is viviparous liberating embryos in successive batches for a period of 3 weeks until the gravid worm completely empties uterine contents
- Body fluid is toxic and responsible for blister formation if it escapes into the tissue.

Embryos

- These are coiled bodies with rounded heads and long slender tapering tails
- They measure 500 to 750 μ × 15 to 25 μ
- The embryos are set free at the time of porturation when the affected part is submerged in water.

Life Cycle

- *Dracunculus medinensis* completes its life cycle in two host, i.e. man and cyclops
- Man acts as definitive host
- Human become infected by consuming water containing infected cyclop
- On reaching stomach of men cyclops get digested by gastric juice releasing larvae.

- Larvae are migrated through digestive tract and loose connective tissue commonly retroperitoneal where larvae grow into male and female adult forms in 6 months, time after seeking entry in humans
- Male worm fertilizers female and dies. In another 6 month's time fertilized female worm migrates to subcutaneous tissue of parts of the body likely to come in contact with water
- The female fertilized worm liberates embryo in water after coming in contact with water
- In short fertilized female worm takes 1 year to mature in humans
- Now cephalic end of worm comes close to skin likely to be in contact with water, e.g backs of water carriers, arms and legs of washermen, and legs of person involved in filling the containers in step wells or ponds
- Water infact provokes a blister which burst leaving ulcer though which worm is extruded
- Another end of worm along with uterus are ruptured releasing many motile first stage larvae into water. This liberation of larvae continue until entire breed has been discharged
- Larvae move in water with stiff motion briskly coiling and uncoiling the body
- For further development larvae are ingested by certain species of Cyclops
- On reaching midintestine of cyclop (intermediate host) larvae penetrate though soft wall come to coelomic cavity. There they moult twice and develop to infective form in about 2 weeks.

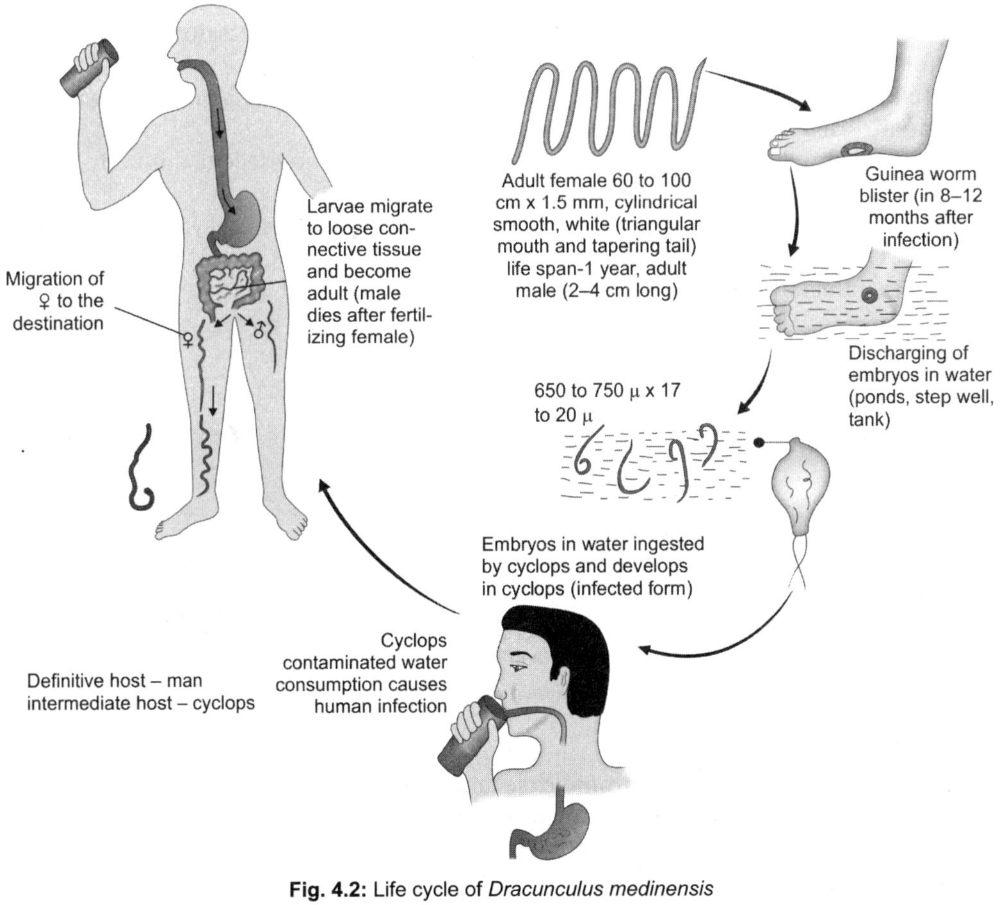

Fig. 4.2: Life cycle of *Dracunculus medinensis*

- Infective larvae seek entry into humans through ingestion or larvae infested water and cycle continues.

Pathogenicity and Clinical Features

- *Dracunculus medinensis* causes dracunculiasis
- Incubation period is about 1 year
- Before appearance of blister infected person may experience, nausea, vomiting, erythema, urticarial rash and prutitis
- There is formation of blisters. The blister fluid is bacteriologically sterile containing lymphocytes, neutrophils, eosinophils and larvae
- Many a time female worm bursts before emergence releasing number of larvae in subcutaneous tissue manifested by intense tissue reaction with formation of abscess
- The blister develops as reddish papule with vascular center and surrounding induration
- The most common sites of blister formation are feet between metatarsal bones or the ankles
- Secondary infection along worm in tissues may occur associated with spreading cellulitis
- Many a time it may result to tetanus.

Laboratory Diagnosis

- Detection of adult worm is possible if worm is dead and calcified. It is done by radiological examination
- Detection of larvae may performed with the help of water. On coming in contact with water larvae are discharged and can be examined microscopically
- Serological test like ELISA, Western Blot and Immunofluoresecent antibody test are beneficial
- Skin test is undertaken with infected dracunculus antigen. There may be appearance of wheal in 24 hours time in infected cases
- Blood examination shows predominant eosinophilia.

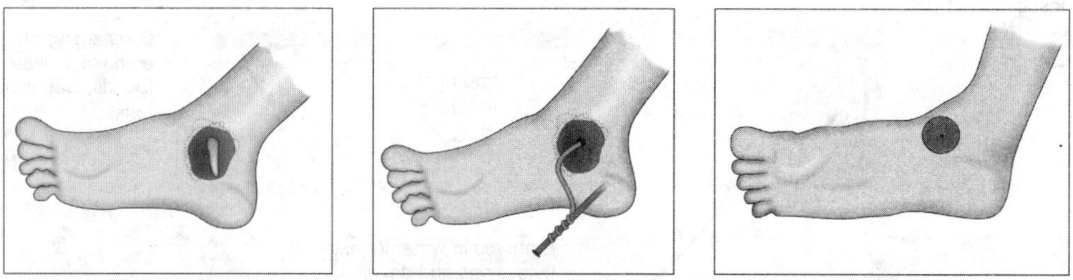

The female guinea worm is protruding through the center of the erosion

An attempt is made to extract the female guinea worm by rolling it around **a stick**

A guinea worm blister, over the medial side of the **right foot**

Fig. 4.3: Extraction of *Dracunculus medinensis* from lesion

Treatment

- Thiabendazole, niridazole, metronidazole, mebendazole and albendazole may hasten expulsion of worm and as antinflammatory agents[3]
- Worms can be removed by twisting adult parasite around a stick. It may take about 20 days to extract whole worm

Prevention

- Filter or properly boil drinking water may be used
- Do not allow infected person to enter the water source
- Treating the water source with insecticide temephos added to pond at the concentration of 1 ppm. It kills cyclops for 5–6 weeks and has low toxicity to mammals and fishes
- Because of preventive measures and active efforts dracunculus has been declared eradicated from Pakistan since 1993 and India since 1997.[4]

FASCIOLA HEPATICA

Synonym

Liver fluke.

History

- *Fasciola hepatica* was the first trematode described in 1379 by de Brie
- It was the first for which the complete life cycle was demonstrated by Leukart and Thomas in 1883 independently of one another.

Geographical Distribution

- Predominant in all sheep rearing and cattle rearing areas like Russia, Europe, Peru, Argentina, Egypt, Iran, Iraq, Northern Thailand, China, Japan, Australia and Africa.[5]
- Infact it has cosmopolitan distribution.

Habitat

The adult *Fasciola hepatica* reside in the biliary passages of the liver of sheep, goat, cattle and human.

Morphology

Adult Worm

- It is large leaf shaped fluke, brown to pale gray in color
- It measure 30 mm × 13 mm
- It is bilaterally symmetrical
- It has no body cavity
- At anterior end there is prominent conical projection, where as posterior end is broadly pointed.
- The oral sucker is situated in conical projection at anterior end and ventral sucker is 1.6 mm
- Intestinal ceca, testes and vitelline follicles of parasite are profusely branched
- Life span of adult worm is 10 years.

Eggs

- They are large, oval, operculate and light yellow brown
- They measure 140 μ × 80 μ
- The shell is thin with smooth surface
- Each egg contains miracidium which extend to the shell margins without clear space.

Life Cycle

- The life cycle of *Fasciola hepatica* needs two hosts to complete life cycle
- Sheep, goat, cattle or human are definitive hosts
- Snail of genus *lymnaea* is the intermediate host
- The eggs are evacuated in the stools of definite host and mature in water
- Miracidium comes out of egg into the water and swims in search of snails an intermediate host
- In snail tissues, it get rid of cilia
- Within 3 weeks of penetration into snail tissues sporocysts start producing first generation radiae (3rd larval stage)
- After 1 week the second generation radiae and ultimately cercariae develop. They come out of snail and swim about in water
- After casting off their tails, they encyst on the blades of grass and other aquatic vegetation
- These are infective forms (metacercae) with grass. Humans get infection by consuming raw vegetables
- Metacercae excyst in duodenum and migrate through intestinal wall into peritoneal cavity
- From here through liver capsule transver set where they settle and grow to maturity. In about a month time, they migrate liver parenchyma to reach biliary passage.
- Adult females liberate eggs through bile to stools. It takes 3–4 months time after actual infection
- The cycle is thus repeated.

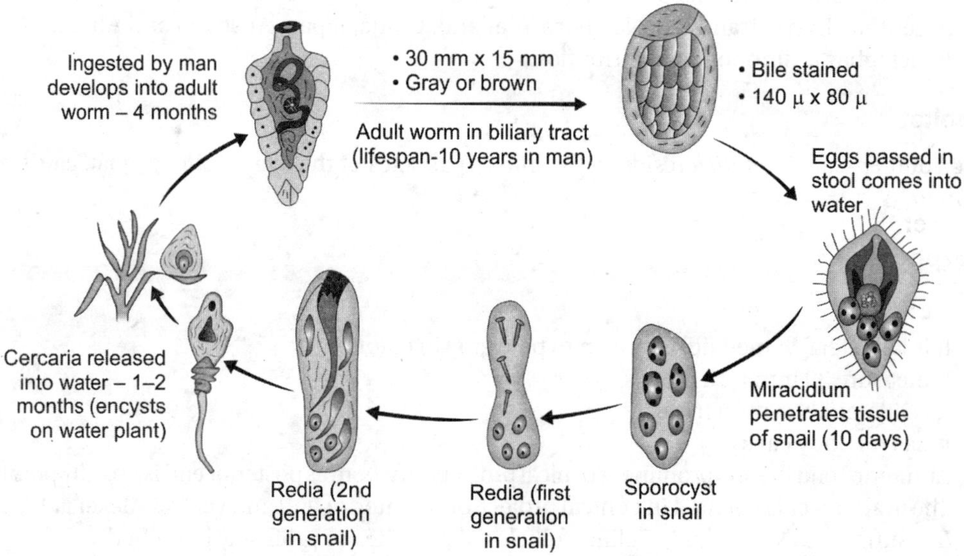

Fig. 4.4: Life cycle of *Fasciola hepatica*

Pathogenicity

- Traumatic and necrotic lesions occur only during migration of larvae through liver parenchyma
- Adult worm in bile ducts provoke inflammatory and edematous changes of biliary epithelium with fibrosis of ducts
- Gallbladder also undergoes pathological changes as happens with bile ducts.

Clinical Features

- Hepatic and obstructive jaundice with coughing and vomiting, generalized abdominal ridigity abdominal tenderness, urticarial, irregular fever, persistant diarrhea, anemia, etc. may occur.
- Cholelethiasis is a frequent complication
- In established infection the manifestations are loss of weight and severe anemia
- Extra biliary fascialiasis may be manifested as dysphagia, dyspnea and even asphyxation. It may be because of inflammation of upper respiratory and digestive tract. Cutaneous manifestations occur in upper abdomen presenting as migrating nodules which are pruritic, painful, inflammed and measure 2–3 cm.

Laboratory Diagnosis

- Detection of eggs in stool or bile obtained by duodenal aspiration
- Eosinophilia which may be moderate to singnificantly high
- Immunodiagnostic tests like ELISA is useful. It is positive in 2 weeks of infection and becomes negative after treatment. CIEP test is also useful
- Antigen from adult worm of this worm gives specific intradermal reaction for *Fasciola hepatica* infection.

Treatment

- Recently hexachloroparaxylene has shown good results in Russia
- Emetine hydrochloride and bithionol may be used with success
- Praziquantel is drug of choice and is given in the dose of 75 mg/kg body weight divided into 3 doses per day for 2 days
- Ectopic flukes may be removed surgically.

Prevention

- Reservoir host may be treated with appropriate drug to eradicate adult worms
- Killing of snails should be executed by using 1:50,000 solution of copper sulfate
- Consumption of raw vegetable should not be permitted.

LARVA MIGRANS

It is human infection with helminth larvae which are actually not adapted to humans. Usually, animal helminths are involved and humans happen to be an abnormal hosts. These larvae are lost in between and keep wandering in abnormal host (human) and are called larva migrans. They are of following two types:

Cutaneous Larva Migrans

This condition is an intense pruritic problem due to prolonged migration of dog and cat hookworms in humans.

History

The first published report of this condition was communicated in 1874 from England.

Etiology

- *Ancylostoma braziliense*
- *Ancylostoma caninum*
- *Nector americanus*
- *Strongyloides stercoralis.*

Transmission

- Actually eggs are developed into filariform larval in optimal environmental temperature and humidity
- In most sandy area, conditions are favorable for development of eggs to larvae and further transmission. These eggs are discharged through stools of infected animals who defecate in moist sandy areas.

Clinical Picture

- Penetration of larvae through skin and their migration is associated with intense itching. Scratching may cause secondary bacterial infection
- In heavy infection the severe itching may leave the patient psychotic.

Laboratory Diagnosis

- Differential leukocytic count may show mild eosinophilia in some of the patients
- Skin biopsy reveals increased eosinophila. However, larvae are hardly observed
- Immune serological tests are not of much use in diagnosing this condition.

Treatment

- Thiabendazole administered orally or applied locally as (0.5 g tablet with 5 g petroleum jelly) is quite effective[6]
- Metriphonate can be given topically as 10% in petroleum jelly and covered with plastic over the worm track and left on overnight
- Advancing part of creeping eruption is frozen with ethylchloride. This has proved quite effective
- In a recent trial a simple 12 mg dose of invermectin has been reported useful rather more effective than 400 mg of albendazole.[7]

Prevention and Control

- Infected dogs and cats should be banned to enter public places like parks and beaches
- Health education regarding avoidance of skin contact with animal fecal contaminated soil
- Visceral larva migrans: It occurs because of migration of parasitic larvae in the visceras of host for prolonged period upto years together.

Etiology

- The commonest causative agent is *Toxocara canis*
- Helminths capable of causing visceral larva migrans include:
  - *Toxocara catis*
  - *Toxocara canis*

- *Angiostrongylus cantonensis*
- *Gnathostoma spinigerum*.

Transmission

- Visceral larva migrans transmission is by ingestion of eggs of *Toxocara* species contaminated edibles or soil
- Usually, children are involved. Children have habit of pica, i.e. eating unnatural things like clay, etc. clay, soil may be contaminated with eggs of helminths.

Pathology

- Primarily liver is involved. Sometimes other organs like lung, heart, kidney, muscles and brain may be involved
- The enlarged liver may show grayish white nodules in the parenchyma. These nodules are made up of eosinophils, Langhans giant cells and larvae. The nodules may be of 2–4 mm in diameter
- In ocular toxocariasis the larvae are seen in the posterior chamber of the eye.

Clinical Picture

- Visceral larva migrans presents the disease in two forms:
  - Visceral form
  - Ocular form
- In visceral form manifestations may be urticarial, asthmatic attacks, weight loss, arthralgia, myalgia, etc. Patient may be suffering from petit mal epilepsy
- In ocular form there is unilateral, painless, solitary lesion in the eye. It may be confused with retinoblastoma leading to wrongly enucleation of the eye. Ocular form is not anyway related to pica.

Laboratory Diagnosis

- Differential leukocytic count shows significant eosinophilia
- Immunoglobulin levels of IgG, IgE and IgA are quite elevated
- Demonstration of larvae in liver biopsy is possible in only 20% cases
- Immunological tests like ELISA using excretory and secretory antigen of second stage larvae of *Toxocara canis* is found equally sensitive and specific. A titer of 1:32 is considered diagnostic.

Treatment

- Diethyl carbamazine is the drug of choice
- Actually treatment is needed when heart, lung, brain, etc. are involved with inflammatory reactions
- Albendazole is reported reasonably effective.

Prevention and Control

- Efforts must be made to reduce environmental contamination due to *Toxocara canis*
- Ingestion of contaminated soil through pica by children must be checked
- Deworming of infective dogs must be done.

REFERENCES

1. Velez LD, Ortega JE, et al. Paragonimiasis in view from Columbia Clin Chest Med. 2002;23:421–31.
2. Toscano, C Hai, YS, et al. Paragonimiasis and tuberculosis diagnostic confusion a review of The literature. Trop Dis Bull. 1995;92:R1–R27.
3. Muller R. Dracunculus and dracunculiasis. Adv Parasitol. 1971;9:73-151.
4. Caircross S, Muller R, Sagaria S. Dracunculiasis (Guinea Worm Disease) and eradication initiative Clin, Microbiol Rev, 2002;15: 223–46.
5. Boray JC, Fascioliasis. In: Hittyer GV, Hopla CE (Eds), Section C, Parasitic Zoonosis Volume CRC Press, 1982,71–88.
6. Harland, PSEG, Meakins RH and treatment of cutaneous larva migrans with local Thiabendazole. BMJ 1977;772 (Letter).
7. Caumes E, et al. A randomized trial of ivermectin versus albendazole of the treatment of cutaneous larva migrans. Am J Trop Med Hyg. 1993;49:641–44.

Schistosomiasis

5

Schistosomiasis is caused by schistosomes. Almost 190 millions persons in over 76 countries in the world are victims and around 652 millions are at risk.[1] Almost 85% of people infected with schistosomes are located in African continent.

The clinical symptoms and pathological changes may reflect migratory routes and host responses to toxic or antigenic substances derived from developmental stage of schistosomes after their penetrating of the skin. Host reaction to eggs laid in vasculature give rise to pathological changes in tissues resulting to granulomas formation. Granulomas promote the egg excretion[2] which is beneficial to parasite. It is useful to host also by effectively isolating, the inflammatory reaction to eggs, thus protecting host tissue adjacent to the granuloma.[3]
Susceptibility to schistosoma infection is present in chromosome 5 q31 to q33. Hepatomegaly in schistosomiasis correlates with expression of specific class I and II histocompatibility antigens. Development of liver fibrosis is related to gene on chromosome 6 q22 to q23, that encodes the receptors of antifibrogenic cytokine interferon gamma.

The drug of choice is praziquantel which is effective against all species of schistosomes. Recently it has been reported that artemether, the methyl ether derivative of artemisinin, is effective against schistosomiasis rather most effective against 7 days old schistomules.[4]

SCHISTOSOMA HAEMATOBIUM

Synonyms

The vesical blood fluke.

History

It was first discovered by Bilharz in 1851 from the mesenteric vein of a native of Cairo, Egypt. It was demonstrated by Bilharz to be the cause of hematuria.[5]

In 1952 cases contacted locally focus was identified by Gadgil and Shah in Ratnagiri district about 140 KM form Mumbai (India) with intermediate host being *Ferrissia tenuis.*[6-8]

Habitat

Adult worms live in pelvic venous plexus (veins surrounding the urinary bladder).

Geographical Distribution

- Prevalent through out the Nile valley and many other parts of Africa
- Middle east and around.

Morphology

- It occurs in two forms adult worms and eggs
- The male adult worm is short and stout measuring 10 to 15 mm × 0.8 to 1 mm. It is covered with minute integumentary tuberculation. It has two suckers of which ventral sucker is larger. The male body is folded all the way to caudal extremity to form gynecophoric canal in which female worm is held during copulation and oviposition
- The female adult worm is long, slender measuring 20 mm × 0.25 mm. The suckers are small and not muscular. Tuberculation is limited to the extremities of the worm
- The adult worm can live upto 25–30 years[6]
- Eggs measure 112 to 170 μ × 40 to 70 μ and they possess distinct terminal spine. Egg shell is transparent and light yellowish brown in color. With every urination act, patient may release 40,000 eggs. Inside egg lies ciliated miracidum.

Life Cycle

- It completes its life cycle in human and fresh water snail
- Humans are definitive host whereas fresh water snails are intermediate hosts usually *Ferrissisa tenuis* in India
- The eggs are discharged through urine of infected person usually toward the end of micturition
- From these eggs ciliated larvae (miracidium—the first larval stage) hatch out in water
- Miracidium comes in contact with intermediate host, i.e. snail. Miracidium penetrate their soft tissues and reach liver and other organs. Miracidium loose their cilia

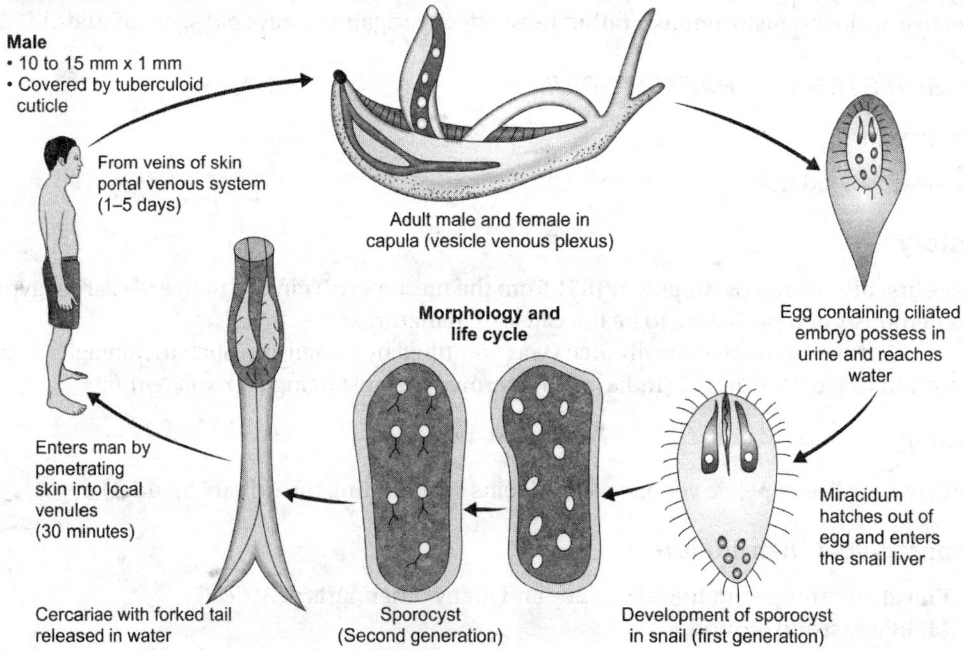

Fig. 5.1: Life cycle of *Schistosoma haematobium*

- In about 8 weeks, miracidium develops first and second generation sporocysts (second stage larval stage) which ultimately are transformed to a generation of fork tailed cercariae. Now they break out of snail in water. They remain viable for a period of 10–25 days.
- When humans happen to take bath in cercariae infested water cercarie come in contact with human skin. The actively motile infective form of furcocercous cercaria cercarae penetrate intact skin. Within the human body they cast off their tail and become schistomules and enter blood stream to reach liver
- In portal vein of humans, schistosomules develop into schistosomes and differentiate into male and female schistosomes. The maturing male and female schistosomes pair migrate to venules of genitourinary plexus. Mature pair mates and gravid female lays eggs. This complete process of development in human may take 2–3 months' time
- The eggs so layed reach urinary bladder to pass in urine especially during afternoon. Eggs hatch in fresh water bodies. The ciliated miracidia possess photoreceptors and they swim in search of snail. Snails live among vegetation in lakes irrigation canals and small collection of water. Thus, life cycle continues
- Pathogenesis
- Metabolites of *Schistosoma hematobium* during development may evoke allergic reactions in the patients
- Granulomatous warty lesions or papultes may appear on the skin over abdomen and around the umbilicus due to presence of adult worm in periumblical plexus
- In urinary bladder, the discharging of eggs may damage wall of urinary bladder and cause hematuria. Moreover infiltration of eggs into tissue may cause fibrosis leading to miliary pseudotubercle formation. This ultimately leads to fibrosis of entire organ. Several mechanisms have been suggested to explain the possible role of *Schistosoma hematobium* in causing malignancy of urinary bladder. They are:
  - Fibrosis induced by schistosoma eggs may induce proliferation hyperplasia and metaplasia
  - Chronic urinary bacterial infection and production of nitrosamines (urinary bladder carcinogen) from percursors in urine may induce cancer[10]
  - Another factor is raised urinary β-glucuronidase from miracidia and adult schistosomes liberating carcinogenic amines in urine[11]
- There may be pseudo abscess formation around the eggs lodged in perivascular tissues
- It has been associated with pancreatic calcification.

Clinical Features

- It causes disease schistosomiasis or bilharziasis
- Cercarial penetration of skin leads to intense irritation and skin rash in 24 hours. It is also called cercarial dermatitis or swimmer's itch which may go away within 2–3 days
- During circulation and maturation of *Schistosoma hematobium* patient may present with fever, cough, lymphadenopathy, hepatosplenomegaly or uriticaria. This condition is called Katayana fever which appears in 4th and 5th week after infection
- Dysuria and hematuria develop 8–12 weeks after infection
- Friable masses are formed in bladder or ureter
- Fibrosis develop may cause complications like hydroureter, hydronephrosis ultimately leading to glomerulonephritis and renal failure

- In certain areas squamous cell carcinoma of bladder is linked with *Schistosoma hematobium infection.*

Laboratory Diagnosis

- Microscopic demonstration of terminal spined eggs in centrifuged deposit of stool
- Demonstration of eggs in biopsied vesical mucosa by compressing biopsy material between slides
- Serological test Cercarian Hullen reaction circumoval precipitation and miracidial immobilization tests detect antibodies against cercariae egg and miracidium respectively. IHA, IFA, ELISA and RIA tests are also used to its diagnosis.

Treatment

- Praziquantel may be administered as single dose of 40 mg/kg body weight. It is drug of choice
- Metrifonate may be given 7.5–10 mg/kg body weight repeated three times at the interval of 2 weeks. Actually it is cheap alternative.

Prevention

- Eradication of snails by molluscides
- Sanitary improvement of environment
- Prevention of pollution of water by infected person
- Avoiding swimming or wading in polluted water
- Health education and sanitary methods to avoid water contamination with urine.

SCHISTOSOMA MANSONI

Synonym

Manson's blood fluke.

History

- Theodar bilharz first reported African schistosomiasis in 1851 but wrongly described that same schistosome lays down two types of eggs (one with terminal spine and other with lateral spine)
- Manson noticed first of all schistosomiasis in New World
- Simbon in 1907 described differences between intestinal and urinary tract schistosomiasis. Simban infact proposed its name manson
- *Schistosoma mansoni* was perhaps introduced in Western hemisphere through African slave trade.

Geographical Distribution

It is common in the Nile Delta, Sudan, the East African coast and in United States (New York).

Habitat

- Adult worms live in mesenteric veins of sigmoidorectal region
- They are also found in the branches of portal veins of liver.

Morphology

- Adult worms are:
  - Male measures 6.4–12 mm and female 7.2–17 mm in length
  - The tuberculation of male worm is more conspicuous and have 6-9 testes
  - In female the ovary is situated at anterior half of the body and uterus is small containing few lateral spined eggs
- Eggs have following features:
  - Have yellow brown transparent shell
  - Bear characteristic lateral spine
  - Measure 114 to 175 μ × 45 to 68 μ
- Miracidum has following characters:
  - Size is larger than that of *Schistosoma hematobium* and *Schistosoma japonicum*
  - Bears larger anterior penetration glands.

Life Cycle

- The definite host is human
- The intermediate host is fresh water snail (*Biomphalaria glabrata* in West Indies, *Biomphalaria pfeifferi* in Africa, *Biomphalaria alexandrina* in Egypt)
- Life cycle resembles with that of *Schistosoma hematobium*.

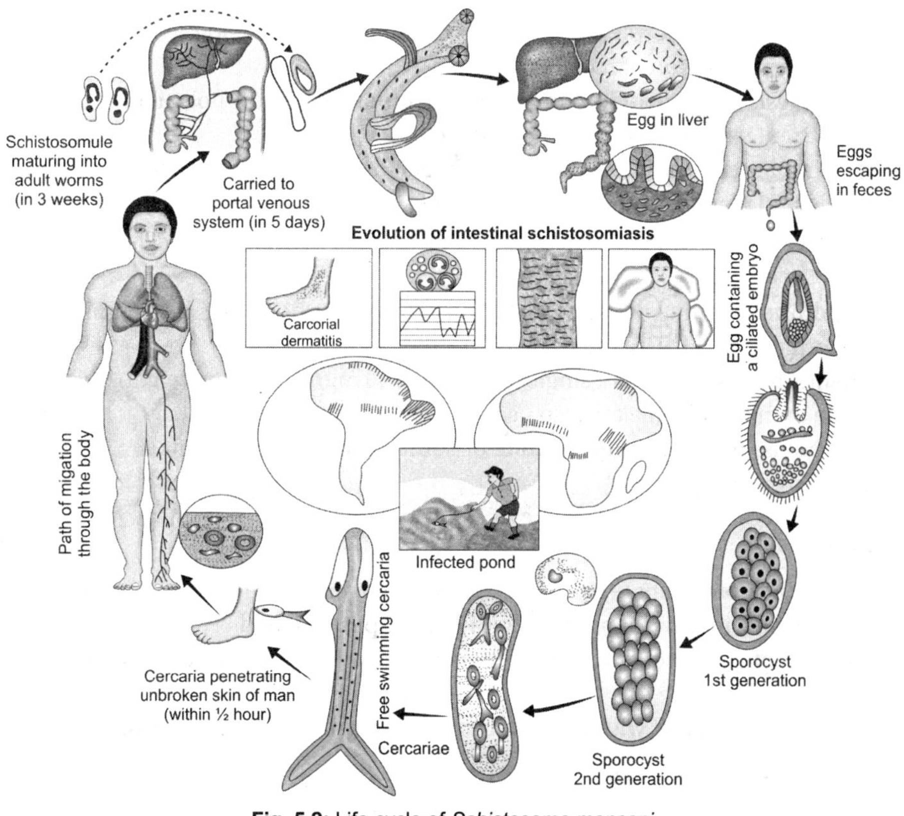

Fig. 5.2: Life cycle of *Schistosoma mansoni*

Pathogenicity

- Katayama fever occurs when infection with this helminth is heavy. In this condition there is fever, lymphadenopathy, hepatosplenomegaly, eosinophilia and elevated immunoglobulin suggesting serum sickness syndrome
- Lesion due to deposition of eggs in colon and appendix (minutes mucosal ulcerating plus hemorrhage)
- Polypoid lesion is seen in rectosigmoid region. There are no edematous lesions
- In liver eggs are found causing granulomatous changes. Liver is markedly enlarged. External surface of liver become uneven. Cut surface of liver shows Symmer's clay pipe stem fibrosis
- Marked splenomegaly
- *Schistosoma mansoni* eggs in appendix may cause obstructive appendicitis.

Clinical Features

- Popular rash with pruritis over skin of the feet
- Dysentery with frequent stool containing eggs
- Incubation period is 7–8 week
- Fever, anorexia, pain abdomen and headache.

Laboratory Diagnosis

- Demonstration of lateral spined eggs from stools using microscope
- Microscopic examination of rectal biopsy is useful
- Serological tests may include complement fixation test slide floeculation tests, ELISA, counter current immmunoelectrophoresis, etc.
- Blood examination in early stages shows leukocytosis with marked eosinophilia. Moderate leukopenia and macrocytosis may develop later.

Treatment

- Oxaminoquine as a single dose of 15–20 mg to 60 mg/kg body weight is administered. Egg count is reduced by 95–97% Cure rate is 70–100%
- Praziquentel may be given as a single oral dose of 40 mg/kg of body weight. Cure rate is 85%
- Niridazole or mebendazole are also useful
- Old drug potassium antimony tartarate or sodium antimony tartarate are still considered effective in treating patients.

Prevention

- Sodium pentachlorophenate has been used with considerable success to control snails
- Patient infected with this helminths should be properly treated
- Construction of public baths, laundry tanks and sanitary drainage canals to control the infection.
- Disinfection of night soil with ammonium nitrate before using it as fertilizer may kill the eggs.

SCHISTOSOMA JAPONICUM

Synonyms

Oriental blood fluke.

History

- The disease schistosomiasis japonica oriental schistosomiasis was mentioned by Fuji a Japanese physician in 1847 in his Katayma memoir
- Fuginami in 1904 first reported the female worm in the portal vein
- Katsurada in 1904 described the adult worm from infected dog cat and man. He described the egg morphology of the parasite *Schistosoma japonicum.*

Geographical Distribution

It is found mostly in China, Japan, Taiwan, Philippines and Indonesia.

Habitat

Adult parasites are found in radicles of superior mesenteric vein draining the small intestine (ileocecal region), also in the intrahepatic portion of portal venous system and rectal plexus of veins.

Morphology

Adult male is 15 to 20 mm × 0.5 mm, covered with minute acuminate spines containing seven testes.

- Adult female is 26 mm × 0.3 mm with ovary lying in the middle of the body. Uterus contains 50 eggs
- Eggs are oval or subspherical 70 to 100 μ × 55 to 65 μ having smooth but thick shell with small lateral knob
- Eggs are discharged through stools.

Life Cycle

- Human, cat, dog, pig or cattle are definite host
- Fresh water snail of genus oncomelania is intermediate host
- Eggs are excreted in stool but require dilution of stool in water to hatch
- Miracidium comes out of egg and starts swimming in water
- It enters soft tissue of snail (*Oncomelania* and *Quadrasi* in the Philippines) and produce first and second generation of sporocysts which develop into fork tailed cercariae
- On contact with human or animal skin the cercariae cast off their tail and penetrate the skin to reach venous circulation
- Schistosomulae pass through right side of heart to lungs then via lungs pulmonary capillaries they reach left side of heart into systemic circulation
- On reaching the intrahepatic portal circulation they feed, grow and migrate into superior mesenteric venules. They grow to adult form and differentiate into males and females. Gravid females lay eggs in mesenteric veinules, penetrate the gut wall and pass through stools. In water the eggs hatch miracidia which are taken up by snail and cycle continues.

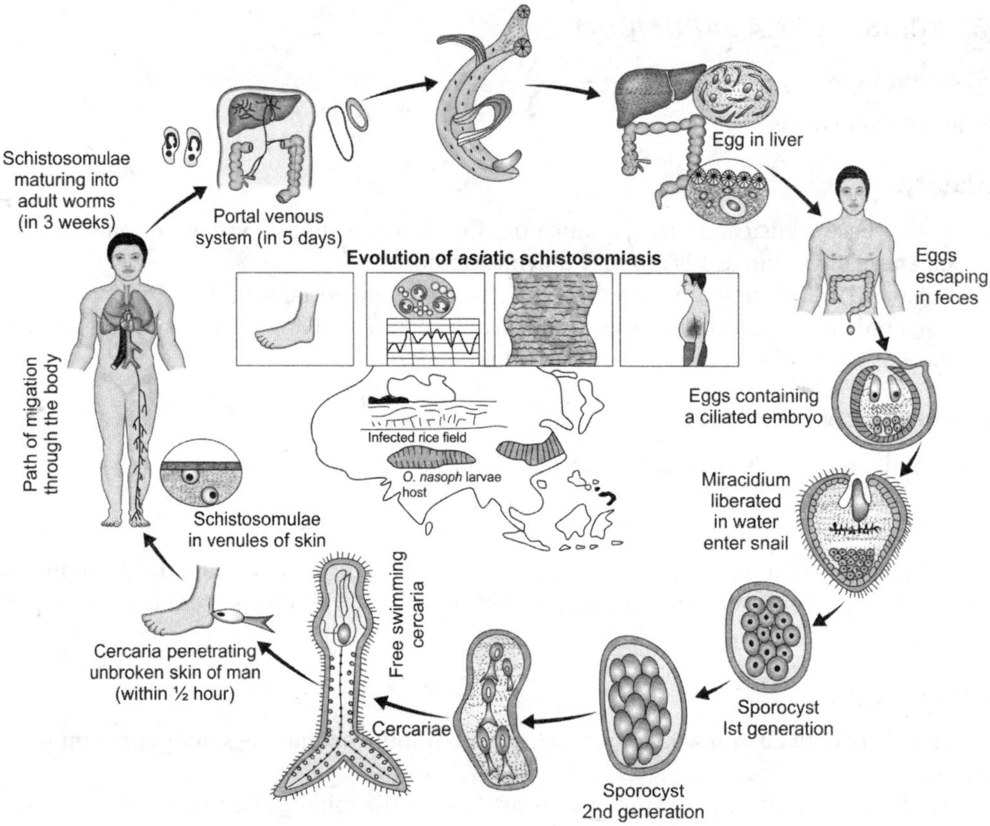

Fig. 5.3: Life cycle of *Schistosoma japonicum*

Pathogenesis

- *Schistosoma japonicum* produces lesions like other *Schistosoma mansoni* and *Schistosoma hematobium*
- Intestinal tract and liver are primarily involved
- The pseudotubercles are formed around eggs and result fibrosis and papillomatous growths.

Clinical Features

- Clinical manifestations are quite severe because of production and liberation of more number of eggs than other schistosome species
- Because of small size of eggs, they are widely disseminated in the body through hematogenous route
- They may involve brain and spinal cord more oftenly
- Eggs may spread to cerebral structures causing epileptic seizures in some patients from Philippines
- In acute stage infection is associated with irritation of skin at the site of cercarial penetration (Swimmer's itch), fever and malaise. Acute infection is quite severe because of *Schistosoma Japonicum* and called Katayama syndrome. Manifestations of Katayama syndrome are high fever, hepatomegaly, lymphadenopathy, eosinophilia and dysentery

- In chronic stage liver shows periportal cirrhosis (Symmer's pipe-stem fibrosis), portal hypertension, esophageal varices and gastrointestinal bleading.

Laboratory Diagnosis

- Detection of eggs of Schistosoma Japonicum in stools
- Detection of eggs from rectal biopsy especially in the situation when eggs are not detected in stools
- Serological tests like ELISA, immunofluorescent antibody, latex agglutination test, complement fixation test, etc.
- Indirect evidences like mucus in blood and eosinophilia.

Treatment

- Potassium antimony tartarate or sodium antimony tartarate happens to be most effective
- Fuadin and anthiomiolin are equally effective
- Praziquantel treatment in intestinal schistosomiasis repeated weekly upto 3 weeks is good. It is markedly effective with low toxicity. Side effects are mild, rare and self limiting. However side effects include abdominal pain, headache, dizziness and skin rashes
- Equally efficient are two antischistosomal drugs, i.e. metrifonate and oxamninquine.

Prevention and Control

- Proper disposal of night soil
- Treatment of night soil with ammonium nitrate to kill eggs before it is used as fertilizer
- Destruction of snails by molluscicides
- Avoiding bathing and wading with polluted water
- Control and preventive measures for reservoir hosts (cats, pigs, buffaloes and wild rat). They constitute an vital handicap to control *Schistosoma japonicum*.

REFERENCES

1. Engel D, Chitsulo L. The global epidermioloigcal situation of Schistosomiasis and new approaches to control and research. Acta Trop 2002:82;139-46.
2. Doenhoft MJ. A role for granulomatous inflammation in The transmission of infections disease. Schistosomiasis and tuberculosis Parasitology, 1997;115:Suppl. S113-25.
3. Sandor M, Weinstock JV. Granilomas in schistosome and mycobacterial infections: a model of local immune responses. Trends Immunol, 2003;24:44–52.
4. Xiao, S.H and Catto, B.A. In virto and in vivo studies of the effect of alremether on schistosoma mansoni, Antimicrobial Agent Chemother, 1989:33:1557–62.
5. Kean BH, Mott KE and Russel AJCeds. Tropical Medicine and Parasitology, Vol,2 Itaca, Cornell. University Press. 1978;475.
6. Gadgie RK, Shah SN. Human schistomiasis in India. Discovery of an endemic focus in Bombay State Indian J Med Sci, 1952; 5:760–63.
7. Sathe BD, Mukerfi S, Gaitonde BB an dRenapurkar DM. Reinvestigation of an old focus of schistosomiasis in Gimvi Village Bull Haffkine Inst. 1981;9:34–37.
8. World Health Organization. 13-22. Nov. 1985, Weekly Epidemiol Res. 1985;60:43.
9. Brand KG Schistosomiasis cancer etiological consideration. Acta. Trop. 1979;36:203–14.
10. Hicks RM, Ismael MM, Walters CL, et al. Assocation of bacteria and urinary nitrosamine formation with schistosoma hematobium infection in the Qualyub area of Egypt Trans. R Soc Trop Hyg. 1982;76:519-28.
11. Lucas SB. Squamous cell carcinoma of bladder and schistosomiasis. East Afr Med J. 1982;59:345-51.

Echinococcosis (Hydatid Disease)

6

ECHINOCOCCOSIS HYDATIDOSIS

Two entities ragarding hydatidosis are common as well as important. They are *Echinococcus granulosus* and *Echinococcus multilocularis* responsible of hydatid disease in humans. *Echinococcus granulosus* may give rise to disease name cystic hydatid disease where as *Echinococcus multilocularis* may cause alveolar hydatid disease.

Infection with Echinococcus in definitive host and intermediate hosts occur worldwide. European form[1] as it is known as has universal distribution. This form is prevalent in many rural areas of the world. Another form, i.e. northern form is encountered in northern parts of North American continents and Euriasia.

Echinococcus multilocularis occurs only in Northern hemisphere. There is apparently an expansion of this original focus since this parasite has been reported in the states of Illinois Nebraske,[2] South Dakota and even a far south as South Carolina.[3]

The Asian areas with *Echinococcus multilocularis* include Turkey, Afghanistan, Iran, India, China and Japan. One of the best overview on hydatidosis is depicted in WHO guidelines.[4]

ECHINOCOCCUS GRANULOSUS

Synonym

Tenia echinococcus.

History

- Hydatid or water cyst in man was known and described since the time of Hippocrates.
- *Echinococcus granulosus* adult worm in the intestine of dog was described by Hartmann first of all in 1685.
- Scolices of larvae were described first by Goeze in 1782.

Geographical distribution

- Commonly found worldwide in cattle and sheep raising areas
- More common in temperate climate
- It occurs in South West Asia, South East Asia and Mediterranean countries.

Habitat

- Man harbors larval form in liver and lungs in particular
- Adult worms are encountered in the small intestine of dogs and other canine animals

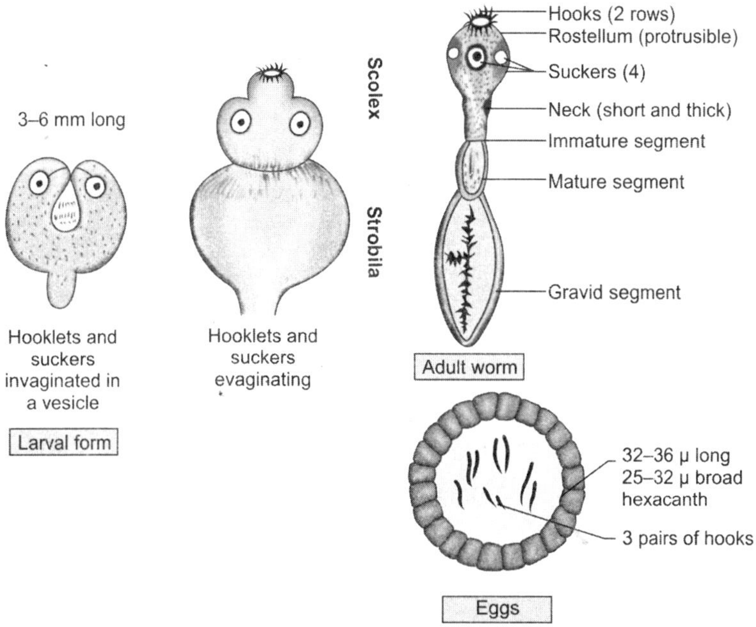

Fig. 6.1: Morphology of *Echinococcus granulosus*

Morphology

Adult worm

- It measures 3 mm to 6 mm in length
- The scolex is small 250 to 500 μ in diameter. It has four deeply cupped oval suckers
- Rostellum is median apical, club shaped refractile armed with 1-7 rows of hooklets
- The neck of worm is short and slender
- The strobila contains 200 proglottides
- Each proglottid may be provided with double set of reproductive organs. Genital pores lie on each lateral margin
- Gravid uterus is sac like and breaks up into many egg capsule enclosed in embryonic membrane containing 8-15 eggs.

Eggs

- They are spherical measuring about 25-40 μ in diameter
- Shell is brick red in color, thin and hyaline, which encloses inner embryophore
- They have fully developed onchosphere with three pairs of hooklets which are present within embryophore
- The eggs are excreted in stools of dogs and can remain viable for 6-12 months in soil
- The eggs are infective to humans, cattles, sheep, etc.

Larval Form

- Larval form can be visualized within hydatid cyst in various organs of intermediate hosts (sheep, cattle, human, etc.).

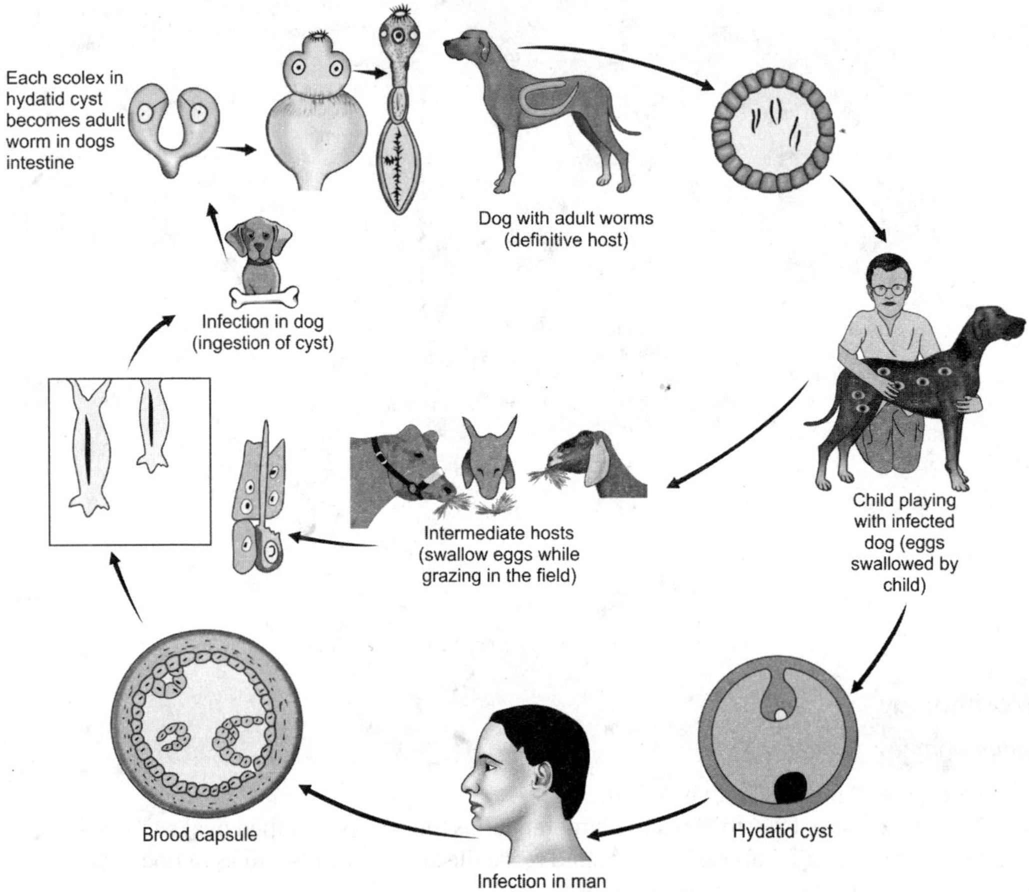

Fig. 6.2: Life cycle of *Echinococcus granulosus*

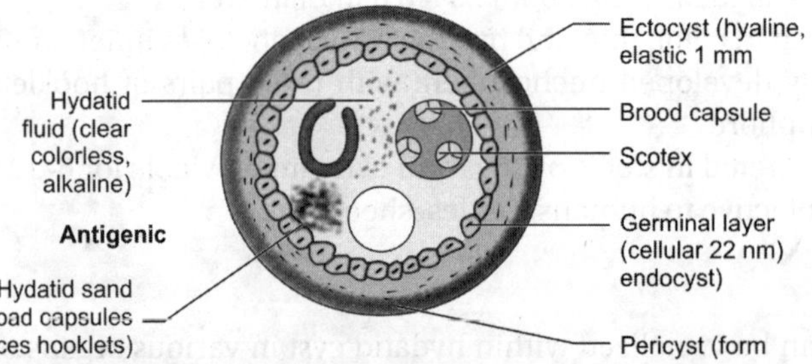

Fig. 6.3: Morphology of Hydatid cyst

- It represents the scolex of future adult worm.
- After entering definite host, scolex along with suckers and hooklets exvaginate and develop into adult form.

Life Cycle

- Dog, wolf, jackal and fox may act as definite host. Adult worm lives in small intestine and liberates number of eggs through stools
- Intermediate host may be human sheep, goat, pig, horse, cattle, etc.
- The eggs are discharged through the feces of definite host
- These eggs are swallowed by intermediate host while grazing in the field
- By coming in contact directly with infected dogs or by permitting dogs to feed from same edibles and water, man may be infected. Man can also acquire infection by consuming edible or water contaminated with egg of *Echinococcus granulosus*
- On reaching duodenum of human hexacanth embryos hatch out of eggs after about 8 hours after ingestion
- The liberated oneosphere penetrate mesenteric blood vessels and are carried to various organs
- Liver acts as first filter and lungs the second filter
- A few embryos may enter general circulation and may lodge in any of the organ of the body
- Wherever embryo succeed to settle, hydatid cyst is formed. Hydatid cyst is surrounded by fibrous tissue and nutrition is supplied to growing embryo through this layer. This layer is known as pericyst and it is not this part of hydatid cyst.
- From inner side of cyst, brood capsule with number of scolices develop
- The mature hydatid cyst may be eaten by dog and other canine animals. It may grow into adult worms. Eggs are layed which are discharged though stools. This way cycle is repeated.

Pathogenicity

- It causes hydatidosis commonly named as hydatid cyst in man
- Infact it is larval form of parasite
- Generally hydatid cyst disease is acquired during childhood but manifestations develop in adulthood
- Hydatid cyst is two layered actually secreted by embryo:
  - Ectocyst is outer layer and is tough acellular laminated and hyaline membrance upto 1mm thick. It is like white of hard boiled egg. When excised or get ruptured it curls on itself (because of elasticity) exposing inner layer having brood capsule, scolices and daughter cysts
  - Endocyst is germinal layer also called inner layer. This layer is comprised of number of nuclei embedded in protoplasmic mass. This layer is about 22–25 μ in thickness. It forms ectocyst on outside and brood capsule and scolices on inside. On breaking free from membrane, embryos float freely in the fluid inside cyst. It is called hydatid sand. It also produces hydatid fluid
- Haydatid fluid secreted has following characteristics:
  - It is clear colorless or pale yellow
  - It specific gravity is 1.005 to 1.1010
  - It is a little bit acidic (pH 6.7)

- It contains sodium chloride, sodium sulphate, sodium phosphate and sodium and calcium salts of succinic acid
- It is antigenic and when absorbed may cause anaphylactic shock. Since it is antigenic, hydatid fluid may be used in Casoni's test
- On centrifugation, deposit (hydatid sand) is obtained which contains brood capsule, free scolices and hooklets

- Acephalocysts formation: Brood capsule and scolices are not formed and hydatid cyst so formed are called ancephalocysts. Infact these cysts are sterile and on ingestion by definite host do not produce infection
- Endogenous daughter cyst:
  - Detachment of fragment of germinal layer may develop into daughter cyst inside mother cyst. This cyst is named as endogenous daughter cyst.
  - Endogenous daughter cyst may contain both ectocyst and endocyst along with brood capsule and scolices
  - Formation of cyst in daughter cyst may be named as grand daughter cyst
- Exogenous cyst:
  - In case of hydatid cyst of bone because of high intracystic pressure rupture of germinal or laminated layer through weaker part of bone may occur. It may result into formation of exogenous cyst

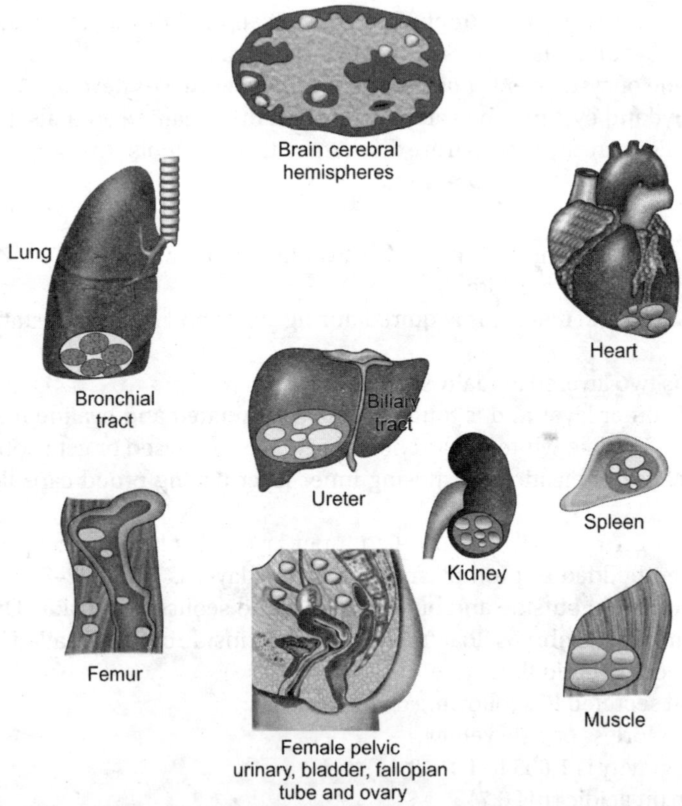

Fig. 6.4: Hydatid cyst of various organs

- The commonest site of hydatid cyst is liver (50–70%) followed by lungs (20–30%). The other sites are spleen, kidneys, heart, bone brain and so on
- The cyst grows very slowly. It becomes 3 mm in size after 3 weeks and 1 cm in 5 months. 80% of the cysts may remain non-viable upto 60 years or more.

Fate of Hydatid Cysts

- Spontaneous recovery in some cases as scolices may die off and fluid may be absorbed slowly
- The cyst may get calcified after the damage to its wall
- As a result of inflammatory reactions spontaneous evacuation of cyst may occur
- Rupture of hydatid cyst of liver may occur into lungs causing disseminated hydatid lesions
- In case rupture occurs in body cavity, there may be widespread of hydatid cysts
- Hydatid cyst rupture may result into anaphylactic shock. Allergic phenomena is quite frequent.[5]

Clinical Features

- Signs and symptoms actually depending upon the location of cyst
- Most of the time it is asymptomatic
- In case of involvement of liver, there may be enlargement of liver
- Rupture of hydatid cyst may lead to allergic signs and symptoms
- Involvement of lungs may give rise to chest pain, cough, dyspnea and hemoptysis
- Cerebral hydatid cyst may produce focal epilepsy and in case of kidney there may be hematuria.

Laboratory Diagnosis

- Blood test: peripheral blood film show moderate eosinophilia in may patients
- X-rays imaging techniques:
  - Plain X-rays permit the detection of hydatid cyst in the lungs. Only calcified cysts may be spotted at other locations
  - CT scan is most specific method to spot hydatid cyst. However, extrahepatic abdominal cysts are not diagnosed definitely with CT scan
  - Radioisotopic, ultrasound and angiography are other methods to diagnose hydatid cyst
  - Recently magnetic resonance imaging (MRI) has proved quite promising
- Detection of scolex in stool, sputum or vomitus is possible in case of rupture of cyst into bile duct, intestine, or bronchus. Hence hooklets may be demonstrated from stool, sputum or vomitus
- Exploratory cyst puncture may reveal presence of proscolices (hydatid sand). However it is not indicated because cystic products may cause anaphylaxis and secondary dissemination of hydatid infection
- Serological tests: The source of antigen include sterile hydatid fluid procured from sheep or man cyst wall or proscolices. This antigen is 8 and 16 kDa antigen. Following test may be performed:
  a. Antibody detection like ELISA, Dot ELISA, indirect immunofluorescence test, latex agglutination test, indirect hemagglutination are useful. In addition precipition test and complement fixation test are also useful. Diagnostic positivity of these tests

varies from 60–90%. The specificity of these tests is based on detection of antibody to Echinococcus antigen 5 (capron's arc 5). Experimental studies indicate that antibodies to antigen 5 are among the first detectable antibodies after infection[6]. Hydatid antigen dot immunoassay is a newer method introduced to diagnose hydatid cyst. Here serum sample is incubated with textile colloidal dye and a nitrocellolose stick to which hydatid antigen has been bound. The presence *Echinococcus* specific antibodies leads to dying of stick reactive area and a color spot develops

b. Antigen detection is possible using double diffusion and countercurrent immunoelectrophoresis techniques. It may be employed to detect specific antigen in sera and cerebrospinal fluid in patient with cerebral hydatid cyst.

- Casoni's test:
  - It was introduced by Casoni in 1911
  - It is based on principle of immediate hypersensitivity
  - The antigen is colleceted from hydatid fluid produced from animal or human cysts and is sterilized by Seitz or membrane filteration
  - The sterilized hydatid fluid (0.2 ml) is infected intradermally on one forearm (anterior aspect) and equal volume of normal saline as a control on other fore arm
  - In positive test a large wheal with multiple pseudopodia around 5 cm in diameter are formed. It happens within 30 minutes on test site. They fades away in 60 minute time.
  - It is sensitive test (55–70%) but not specific test.
- Histological examination reveals different layers of surgically removed hydatid cyst. The layers are pericyst ectocyst and endocyst.
- Hydatid disease of liver may be differentiated from hepatoma on the basis of following tests:
  - Serum glycoproteins levels
  - Serum aminotransferases levels
  - Other liver function tests
  - ESR

All above tests are normal in hydatid disease and abnormal in hepatoma. However, ESR is moderately evevated in hydatid disease whereas in hepatoma it is markedly elevated.

Treatment

- Surgical removal of hydatid cyst. It is preferred treatment when cysts are more than 10 cm in diameter. The cyst must be removed in toto and strict precautions must be taken to avoid spilling
- It is a must to use scolicidal agents. Currently used scolicidal agents include, chlorohexidine, hydrogen peroxide, ethanol and cetrizamide[7,8]
- Pretreatment with benzimidazole compound is proposed to avoid the use of dangerous scolicidal agents[9] and to decrease the rate of recurrence[10]
- After radical surgery chemotherapy should be given for minimum 2 years to avoid recurrence.
- Mebendazole and albendazole are active against *Echinococcus granulosus* as they penetrate into cyst and are quite effective
- Albendazole is preferred as its bioavailability is better. It is given in cycle of 4 weeks followed by a drug free interval of 2 weeks. Dose per day varies 400–800 mg. Success with albendazole varies from 66–100%, In 22% cases hepatic cysts completely disappear.

Prevention and Control

- Strict and personal hygiene
- Dogs should not be allowed to eat carcasses of sloughtered animals
- Check on the population of stray dogs
- Direct contact with infected dogs should be checked
- Water and vegetable contamination should be avoided.

ECHINOCOCCUS MULTILOCULARIS

Synonyms

- Alveolar hydatidosis
- Multilocular hydatid disease.

History

- Virchow in 1855 first recognized a hydatid disease in humans that was different morphologically from that of a typical unilocular hydatid cyst
- Leuckart in 1863 named it as *Taenia echinococcus multilocularis*
- Thomas in 1954 worked out its life cycle.

Geographical Distribution

- Europe
- America
- Canada
- Russia
- Central Asian Republics
- Western China
- India
- Iraq
- Iran.

Morphology

It is found in adult form and egg form.

Adult Form

- It is small in size measuring 1.4–5.4 mm
- Large (28-34μ) and small (23–31) rostellar hooks are present
- Number of proglottides varies from 2–6
- Number of testes is 21–29 where as they are 45–65 in case of *Echinococcus granulosus.*

Eggs

- They are similar to other *Taenia* species
- They resist to cold.

Life Cycle

- Definitive hosts are foxes, wolves, domestic dogs and cats
- Intermediate hosts are squirrels, field mice and voles. Man is however accidental intermediate host
- The adult worm remains attached with mucosa of the small intestine of definitive hosts. The eggs are passed with the stools
- The eggs so passed are infective to intermediate hosts
- Humans acquire infection by ingesting vegetables, fruits, salads contaminated with stool of foxes and dogs, etc.
- When infective eggs are ingested by humans a six hooked larval stage known as oncosphere hatches
- Oncosphere penetrates the intestinal wall, enters the circulation, settles in liver spleen and may be brain
- Where oncosphere settles, alveolar hydatid cyst grows as honeycombed structure.

Pathogenesis

- *Echinococcus multicularis* causes alveolar echinococcosis or multilocular hydatid cyst
- The cyst has multiple locules
- The multilocular infiltrating lesion appears as grossly invasive growth that may be mistaken for malignant tumor
- Destruction of liver perenchyma may cause liver failure
- It may metastasize to lungs and brain
- It is most lethal of all helminthic infections of man
- Central necrosis and cavitation are main findings. Cavities contain little or no fluid
- Hyaline layer formed in thin and unconspicous
- Germinal layer is hyperplasitc and folded on itself. There is tendency of persistent follicular reaction by eosinophils and endothelial cells in surrounding tissues
- These multilocular hydatid cysts in man are sterile.

Clinical Features

- Incubation period may be upto 30 years
- Symptoms include pain in right upper quadrant of abdomen and palpable liver
- Because of portal hypertension hepatic cirrhosis may develop
- Enlargement of liver with jaundice may be there
- When metastasis occur in brain or lungs, symptoms of space occupying lesion may develop.

Laboratory Diagnosis

- Diagnosis of this condition may be made by taking biopsy of involved organ. There is rarely presence of scolices. However, characteristic germinal layers and laminated membrane identification help in diagnosing this disease
- Radiology and ultrasound will reveal a solid, space occupying lesion
- CT scan may be helpful in ascertaining site and shape of cyst
- Serological tests are useful by making use of Em1 and Em2 antigen (obtained from metacestodes of *Echinococcus multilocularis* containing specific glycolipids). These antigens may be used in differentiating *Echinococcus granulosus* and *Echinococcus multilocularis.*

Antibodies against specific *Echinococcus multilocularis* (Em2) antigen can be detected with the help of monoclonal antibodies by ELISA and thin layer chromatography
- Newer tests helpful include recombinant *Echinococcus multilocularis* antigen hybrid test and PCR tests, etc.

Treatment

- Surgical removal of cyst is actually difficult because of limiting membrane. Hence entire hepatic area is resected. In fact surgical excision is rarely possible and disease is usually fatal
- Administration of albendazole and mebendazole (40 mg/kg body weight) may cause improvement if given for 3 years
- Since interferon alfa and interferon gamma levels are decreased in patients suffering from this condition so addition of interferon gamma with mebendazole is reported to check the disease progression.

Prevention and Control

- Education and proper personal care
- Deworming of farm dogs and cats
- Treatment of infected animals
- Proper washing of fruits before consuming.

REFERENCES

1. Eckert J, Gemmell MA, Meslin FX, et al. WHO/OIE manual on Echinococcosis in humans and animals; a Public Health Problem of Global Concern, Paris; WHO/OIE, 2001.
2. Ehrhardt AR, Reuter S, Buck AK, et al. Assessment of disease activity in alveolar echinococcosis: a comparision of contrast-enhanced ultrasound, three phase helical CT and (18)F fluorodeoxyglucose positron-emission tomography, Abdom Imaging 2006 Dec2: [Epub ahead of print].
3. Williams DE, Williams GA, Caya JG, et al. intraocular *Echinococcus multilocularis*. Arch Ophthalmol 1987;105:1106–09.
4. Strohmaier WL, Bicher KH, Wilbert DM, et al. Alvoelar echinococcosis with involvement of the ureter and tests. J Urol. 1990;144:733-34.
5. Werezberger A, Colhman J, Wertheim G, Gunders AE, Chowers J. Dissemianated echinococcosis with repeated anaphylactic shock. Chest, 1979;74:482-84.
6. Conder GA, Anderson FL Schantz PM. Immunogianosis tests for hydatidosiss in evaluation of double diffusiojn, immunoelectrophoresis, indirect hemagglutination and intradermal test. J Parasitol. 1980;66:577–84.
7. Schaefer JW, Khan MY. Echinococcosis (Hydatid disease) lesions from experience with 59 patients. Rev Infec Dis. 1991;13:243-47.
8. Langer JC, Rose DB, Keystone JS, Taylor BR, Langer B. Diagnosis and management of hydatid disease of the liver. A 15 years North American experience. Ann Surg. 1984;119:412–17.
9. Morris DL. Preoperative albendazole therapy for hydatid cyst. Br J Surg. 1987;74:805–06.
10. French CK. Mebendazole and surgery for human hydatid disease in Turkana. East Afr Med J 1984;61:113–19.

7 Filariasis

Filariasis is caused by vector borne tissue dewelling nematodes called filariae. Adult may live in lymphatics, blood vessels, skin connective tissues or serous membranes depending upon species of worm involved. Microfilariae are liberated by female adult worm. The microfilariae may live in bloodstream or skin. All true filariae causing infection in human, e.g. Onchorcercideae are transmitted by dipteran vector. The transmission of human filariae is mostly limited to warm climate. High temperatrure is necessary for parasite to develop in vector.

The infective form of the parasite is third stage larva which may be transmitted by vector. The rate of growth, life cycle, differentiation of worms longevity of microfilariae and adult worms differ widely between different species. The life span of some adult worm may extend upto 20 years even.

Onchocerciasis and lymphatic filariasis are quite significant infections. Dracunculiasis may cause ulceration and calabar swellings. Loasis may result to other manifestation leading to severe consequent to the patients.

WUCHERERIA BANCROFTI

Synonyms

- Filaria sanguinis hominis.
- Filaria bancrofti.
- Wuchereria pacifica.

History

- Filariasis has been known since antiquity
- Elephantiasis as a matter was described in India by Sushrata
- The term malbar leg was used to the condition by Clarke in 1709 in Cochin (India)
- Microflaria was identified first of all in 1863 in a patient in his hydrocele fluid
- Brazilian physician Wucherer reported microflaria in chylous urine in 1866. The name of genus is after this great research scholar
- Vector of this parasite, i.e. culex mosquito and its role in the transmission of disease was reported first of all by Manson in 1878
- The name filaria bancrofti was proposed by Cobbold in 1877.

Geographical Distribution

- Asia
- Africa

- Australia
- South Africa.

Habitat

- Adult worms live in lymphatics of lymph nodes of humans.
- Sheathed microflaria are found in blood.

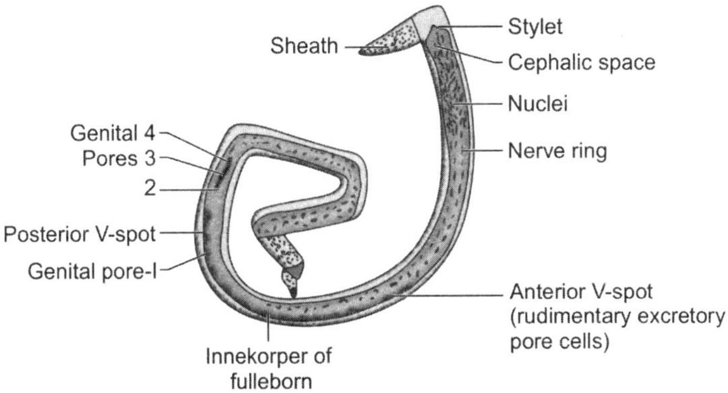

Fig. 7.1: Microfilaria of *Wuchereria boncrofti*

Morphology

- *Wuchereria bancrofti* exists as adult and microfilarial forms
- The adult worms are thread like and live in lymphatic tissues of human as tightly coiled nodular masses. Their ends are rounded and lined by smooth cuticle. Adult male worm measure 35 to 40 mm × 0.1 mm whereas adult female worm is 90 mm to 100 mm × 0.25 mm. Life span of adult worm is 3 to 5 years. Female worm liberates sheathed embryos (microfilaria)
- Microflariae of this parasite live in blood vessels. They are actively motile and are encountered in peripheral blood between 10 PM and 4 AM. They measure with hyaline sheath which is a little longer about 35 μ long. Head end of microfilaria is somewhat blunt and tail end is tapering. In unstained preparation microfilariae are colorless and transparent. On staining with Giemsa or Romanowsky, they are visualize as pink colored with a column of violet nuclei. These nuclei are absent at the head and tail ends. The column of nuclei is broken at places representing primordia of organ like nerve ring, excretory pore, excretory cells genital cells and anal pore
- Microfilariae actually develop in mosquito.

Life Cycle

- Humans are definite host
- Mosquitoes of the genera Culex, Aedes and Anopheles are the intermediate hosts
- Third stage larvae which are found in proboscis sheath of mosquitoes are the infective form in humans
- This infective form of larvae is deposited on the skin of humans at the site of the mosquito bite
- The larvae pass through puncture wound and find way to subcutaneous tissue

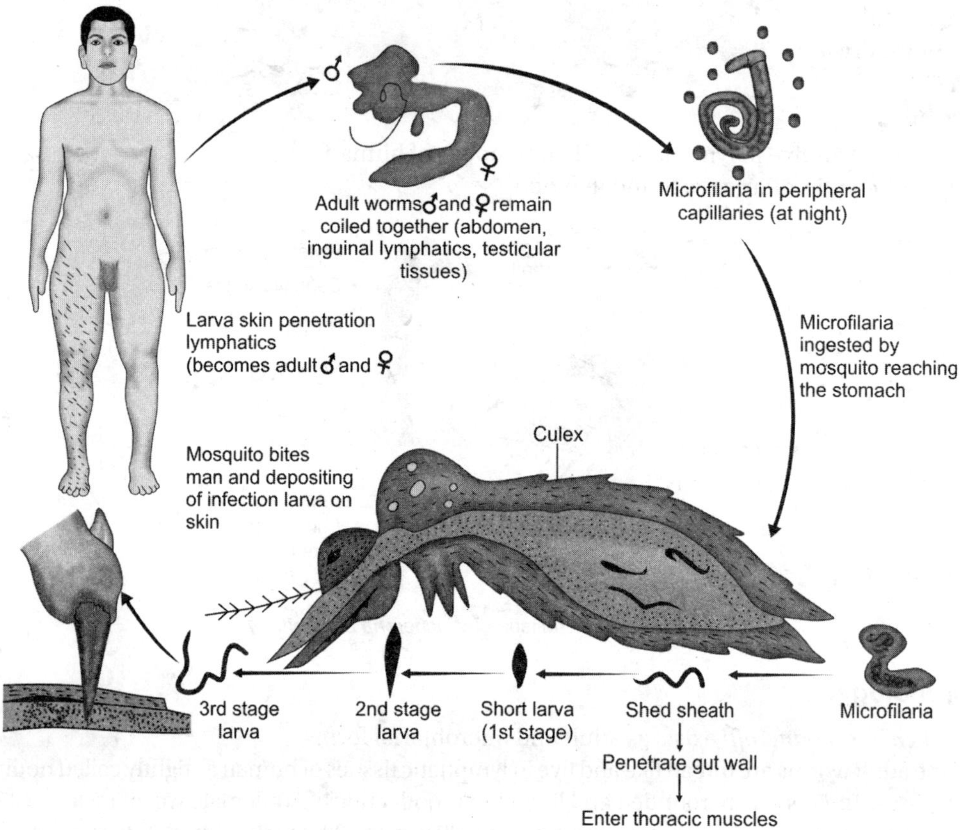

Fig. 7.2: Life cycle of *Wuchereria bancrofti*

- Larvae now enter afferent lymphatics and ultimately reach draining lymph nodes where they develop into adult worm in 3–15 months
- The adult worms differentiate into males and females and may fertilizes female and later gravid female gives birth to sheathed embryo (microfilariae)
- Microfilariae liberated enter efferent lympahtics to enter blood circulation through thoracic duct
- *Wuchereria bancrofti* microfilariae come to peripheral blood between 10 PM and 4 AM. The nocturnal periodically is connected with night biting nature of mosquitoes.
- The sheathed microfilariae are transferred to mosquitoes at the time of mosquito bite with the blood meal
- Now microfilariae lose their sheath in the stomach of mosquitoes and penetrate the gut wall to reach thorax. Now microfilariae develop into first stage, then 2nd stage and ultimately into 3rd stage infective larvae
- The third stage infective larvae measure 1500 to 2000 μ × 18 to 23 μ, enter proboscis and are now ready to infect new host
- Development of microfilariae in mosquitoes may take 7–20 days. However, this duration depends on atmospheric temperature, humidity and species of mosquito
- Multiplication of parasite does not take place in mosquitoes.

Pathogenesis

- In non-endemic areas even small number of microfilariae may evoke immune response and give rise to clinical manifestations.
- Pathological features are due to lymphangitis and lymphadenitis.
- Immune reactions are because of mostly adult worms. The involved lymph nodes and vessels are infiltrated with macrophages, eosinophils, lymphocytes, plasma cell and exhibit endothelial hyperplasia.
- Recently it has been shown that microscopic hematuria occurs in many microfilaremia persons. Levels of eosinophilia is not connected to severity of symptoms.[1]
- In occult filariasis there are no microfilaria in peripheral blood film but patient is symptomatic infact microfilaria are present in lymph nodes and other internal organs, e.g. lungs, liver and spleen.

Cause of Lymphangitis

- Mechanical irritation because of movements of parasites
- Toxic products from dead worms
- Metabolites liberated by growing larvae
- Secondary bacterial infection.

Causes of Lymphatic Obstruction

- Mechanical blockage by dead worms
- Obliterate endolyphangitis
- Fibrosis of lymphatic vessels
- Fibrosis of the lymph node.

Clinical Features

- Infection caused by *Wuchereria bancrofti* is called wuchereriasis or bancroftian filariasis. It may be symptomatic or asymptomatic
- Allergic manifestations include maliase, headache, nausea, vomiting, pruritis, urticaria and fugitive swellings
- Lymphangitis occurs repeatedly accompanied by fever. Lymphatics of testes and spermatic cord may be involved with epididymorchitis and funiculitis
- Filarial fever is usually high fever of sudden on set with rigors. It lasts for 2–3 days. This occurs repeatedly at interval of weeks or months
- Lymphandenitis occur in inguinal lymph nodes and then involving axillary lymph nodes. Swollen lymph nodes are tender and painful too
- Lymphangiovarix is dilatation of lymph vessels involving inguinal, scrotal, testicular or abdominal areas
- Lymphorrhagia is rupture of lymph varices resulting to release of lymph or chyle. It may cause chyluria, chylous diarrhea, chylous ascites and chylothorax
- Hydrocele is due to obstruction of lymph vessels of spermatic cord and exudation from inflamed testes and epididymis
- Lymphedema develops due to successive attacks of lymphangitis. In lymphedema there is swelling against ankle, back of foot and leg. To start with there is pitting edema which later on becomes non-pitting one.

- Elephantiasis: It happens in chronic cases where repeated lymphangitis, obstruction and lymphedema occurs. There is connective tissue hypertrophy and hyperplasia. The part becomes unusual enlarged and surface skin becomes coarse elephantiasis is common in legs, arms, breast, scotum, penis, vulva, etc.
- Occult filariasis is considered due to hyperimmuneresponsiveness against microfilariae. It is also called tropical eosinophilia or tropical pulmonary eosinophilia. Usually it is asymptomatic. Its feature include:
  - High absolute eosinophil count (3000 to 50,000 per cu mm of blood)
  - High titer antibody to filariae
  - High serum level of IgE
  - Nocturnal paroxysmal cough, wheezing and dyspnea
  - Improvement with treatment (DEC)
  - No microfilaria is seen in peripheral blood film.

Laboratory Diagnosis

Diagnosis of *Wuchereria bancrofti* is made as follows:

Demonstration of Microfilaria

- Peripheral blood sample is collected between 10 PM and 4 AM
- Hypereosinophilia is most common feature particular tropical pulmonary eosinophilia. Absolute eosinophil counts range from 3000 to 60,000 cells/mm^3 of blood. However levels of eosinophilia is not related to severity of symptoms
- Unstained film is prepared by taking 2–3 drops of blood on clean glass slide. A clean cover slip is placed over it and sealed with vaseline. Under low power microscope actively motile microfilaria are visualized. By this method microfilaria less than 100 mf/ml are not detectable. Microfilaria are viable for 24–48 hours at room temperature
- Both thick and thin blood smears are prepared on a clean glass slides and dried. With a drop of distilled water thick smear is dehemoglobinized. Now smear is stained with Leishman, Giemsa and polychrome methylene blue stain. Microfilaria are seen microscopically (low power)
- Concentration techniques are quite useful especially if there is low level infection. Commonly used techniques are:
  - Knott's
  - Membrane filtration
  - Saponin lysis
- DEC provocation method is quite advantageous. A small dose of DEC provokes the microfilaria to appear in peripheral blood even during day time. DEC is administered in the dose of 2 mg/kg body weight as a single dose. Blood sample is collected about one hour after for detection of microfilaria
- Microfilaria can be demonstrated from clinical samples like lymph, chylous, urine, hydrocele fluid, exudate of lymph varix, etc.
- Microfilaria are not found in following conditions:
  - Occult filariasis
  - Lymphatic obstruction
  - Early allergic symptoms.

Demonstration of Adult worm

- Adult worm can be demonstrated in lymph node biopsy
- Calcified worm is detected on X-ray examination.

Immunodiagnosis

ELISA, IHA, IFA are useful for detection of filarial antigen. Here monoclonal antibodies against microfilarial larval surface antigen are used.

DNA Probes

DNA probes have been developed for *Wuchereria bancrofti.*

Treatment

Diethylcarbamazine remains the drug of choice for treatment of bancrofti filariasis. It is administered orally in the dose of 6 mg/kg body weight daily for 12 days. It actively kills microfilaria. However, heavy doses may kill adult worms

Prevention and Control

- Eradication of vector mosquito
- Detection and treatment of carriers
- Open drains, septic tanks, soakage pits and flood pit latrines should be taken care of properly.

BRUGIA MALAYI

Synonym

Wuchereria malayi

History

Brug in 1927 described a new microfilaria in the blood of natives of Sumatra. The genus brugia was named after this research scholar.

Geographical Distribution

It occurs in:

- India
- Indonesia
- Philippines
- Malaysia
- Thailand
- Vietnam
- Japan
- China
- South Korea.

In India it is found in:

- Kerala
- Assam

- Odisha
- West Bengal
- Madhya Pradesh.

Habitat

- The adult worm inhabits in lymphatic vessels and glands
- Sheathed microfilaria occurs in blood.

Morphology

- They are smaller in size
- It occurs in adult form and microfilaria form.

Microfilaria

- Microfilaria measures 220 to 250 μ × 6 μ
- With Giemsa stain it looks deeply stained
- Body curves are irregular and twisted
- Cephalic space is almost twice as long as broad
- Stylet at anterior end is double
- Excretory pore is prominent
- Body nuclei are coarse and overlapping
- One can visualize two distinct tail tip nuclei, one at the tip and other one as subterminal.

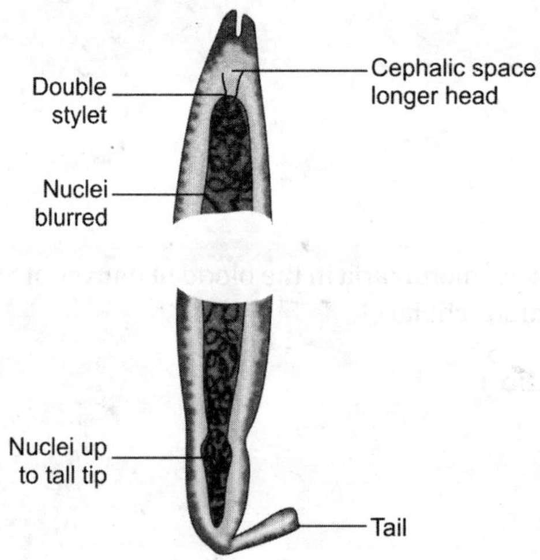

Fig. 7.3: Microfilaria of *Brugia malayi*

Life Cycle

- It resemble *Wuchereria bancrofti*
- Vector is mansonia
- Vector in India is *Mansonia annulifera*
- Microfilaria is nocturnal.

Clinical Picture

- It is almost same as produced by *Wuchereria bancrofti.*
- Prenental sensitization of fetus by infected mothers has been demonstrated to occur in human lymphatic filariasis[3]
- It is slightly different than *Wuchereria bancrofti,* because it rarely causes genitalia elephantiasis.

Diagnosis

- Many techniques are described for demonstrating microfilariae in blood samples. The counting chamber technique is fast, quantitative and cheap.[4] Recently developed parasitological techniques are:
  - Techniques for preserving blood specimens for membrane filtration[5]
  - Techniques for staining of microfilariae sheath in thick, blood smear with fluroscence conjugate lectin for rapid detection of microfilariae[6]
  - The use of microhematocrit tube technique using acridine orange in the tube[7]
- Cross reaction of serodiagnosis tests have been reduced through detection of specific IgG and IgE antibodies[9]
- Monoclonal based antibody based tests for circulating antigen show encouraging result in the diagnosis of filarial infection.[10,11]

Treatment

DEC is the drug of choice.

Prevention and Control

Removal of Pistia plant which is the site of *Mansonia annulifera* breeding. It helps to control vector.

LOA LOA

Synonym

The eye worm.

History

The *Loa loa* worm extracted from the eye of a Negress in St Domingo, West Indies in 1770.

Geographical Distribution

It is predominant in central and western parts of tropical Africa.

Habitat

- Adult worms live in subcutaneous connective tissues of humans
- Quite oftenly adults are also found in subconjunctival tissue of the human eye
- The sheathed microfilaria are detected in the blood.

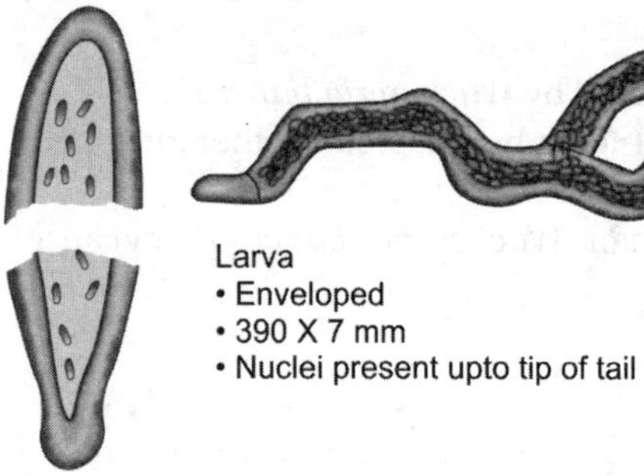

Fig. 7.4: Microfilaria of *Loa loa*

Morphology

Adult Worm

- Adults are thin, whitish and taper toward cephalic end
- Male measures 30 to 35 mm × 0.35 to 0.42 mm
- Female is 40 to 70 mm × 0.5 mm in size
- The caudal end of male is curved ventrally and bears narrow alae
- The vuvla opens in female in cervical part
- Its life span is 17 years or more.

Microfilariae

- By and large microfilariae of *Loa loa* resemble with *Wuchereria bancrofti, Brugia malayi* except that column of nuclei extends completely to the tip of tail
- The sheath in the microfilaria extends beyond the anterior and posterior end of the larvae
- It measure 250 to 300 μ × 6 to 8 μ
- It exhibits diurnal periodicity with maximum microfilaria at mid day.

Life Cycle

- Life cycle is completed in two hosts, i.e. man and day biting female mango fly (chrysops dimidiata, chrysops siliacea)
- Female infected chryosops bite human and infective larvae enter through punctured skin made by vector during bite
- Now larvae find way in subcutaneous tissue, moult and grow to mature adult worms
- They differentiate into male and female worms
- Male worm fertilizes female who produce microfilariae which circulate in peripheral blood during day time. Ultimately, they enter in subcutaneous tissue
- The optimum site for microfilaria during non-circulation phase is the lungs
- The sheathed microfilaria are ingested by female chrysops during blood meals. They cast off sheaths and penetrate stomach wall reach thoracic muscle where they grow to infective larvae. It takes 10 days to complete life cycle in chryosops
- The mature infective larval migrate to mouth parts of chryosops for onward transmission to human hosts and cycles goes on.

Pathogenicity

- Most of clinical symptoms are due to allergic reactions to the worms resulting in the formation of swelling called calabar swellings. Calabar swelling measure 3–10 cm
- The worm can also be seen migrating in subconjunctival tissue (African eye worm)
- Nephropathy, encephalopathy and cardiomyopathy may occur rarely.

Clinical Features

- *Loa loa* produced the disease in man called loasis
- Produced swellings called fugitive or calabar swellings which are painless, edematous last for few hours to few days and reappear elsewhere. They are common on the back of hands or arm.[14] They are because of reactions to waste products of adults or probably microfilariae. These reactions are accompanied by itching, erythema, fever, pruritis with high eosinophilia
- Wondering adult worms reach under the conjunctiva causing discomfort and edema of eyelid.[15] It may also cause granulomata in bulbar conjunctiva and proptosis. Conjunctival granulomatas are solitary or multiple yellow nodules about 2 mm in size.

Laboratory Diagnosis

- Demonstration of microfilaria in peripheral blood film collected during day time (10 AM to 2 PM)
- Isolation and identification of adult worm from the eye or from subcutaneous biopsy
- Eosinophilia and significant levels of antifilarial antibodies especially in presence of calabar swellings
- A PCR assay with high specificity and sensitivity for microfilaremia and occult loiasis has been developed.[16]

Treatment

- Administration of DEC 8–10 mg/kg body weight/day for 21 days
- It is effective against both adult and microfilaria larvae
- In heavy infection it is essential to give glucocorticoids along with DEC to prevent encephalitis and coma
- Adult worm can also be removed surgically. The most favorable time is when worms are migrating through the bridge of the nose.

Prevention and Control

- Protection from chrysops bites by using repellants
- Killing of chrysops
- Identification of patients and treating them with DEC.

ONCHOCERCA VOLVULUS

Synonyms

- Convoluted filaria
- Filaria volvulus

Geographical Distribution

- Tropical Africa
- Central America
- Arabian peninsula (Yemen) in Asia.

Habitat

Adult worms are found in the subcutaneous tissue of human

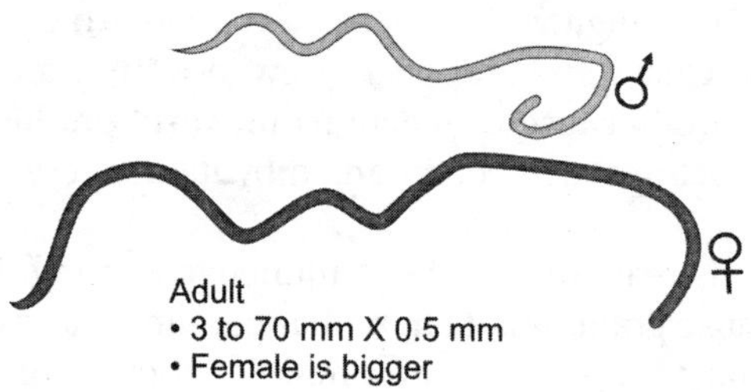

Fig. 7.5: Adult worms of *Onchocercal volvulus*

Morphology

It is found in adult form and larval form.

Adult Form

- It is white opalescent and transparent having transparent striations on the cuticle
- Male is 1.9 to 4.2 cm × 0.13 to 0.2 mm in size with a coiled tail
- Female worm is 33.5 to 50 cm × 0.27 to 0.40 cm in size
- Average life span of adult worm is 8 years and may extend upto 15 years.

Microfilaria

- It measures 240 to 360 μ × 3 to 9 μ
- Nuclei column does not extend to tail tip
- They are unsheathed and non-periodic
- They may be found in lymphatics of connective tissue and corneal conjunctiva.

Life Cycle

- It completes its life cycle in two hosts
- Humans are definitive host
- Day biting female black fly of genus simulium is the intermediate host. This black fly is also called buffalo gnat
- The vector simulium breeds in fast flowing river and the disease occurs commonly along with the course of river and so called river blindness
- Humans are infected by the bite of black fly which carry third stage infective larvae in the mouth parts
- Through punctured wound of skin the larvae enter and migrate to subcutaneous tissue. Here larvae moult twice and develop into male and female adult worm.

- Adult worm may live singly, in coiled entangled masses in subcutaneous tissue or in deep fascia
- Male fertilizes female worm. Fertilized female worm release actively motile, unsheathed microflariae which migrate to the skin and eyes of infected person where they can survive for 1-2 years.
- Now black fly may bite an infected person at one of the infected site. As a result microfilaria are taken up from skin and lymphatics and develop in the black fly. The microfilaria reach gut form where they migrate to thoracic muslces. Here they moult twice and develop into infective larvae in 6–8 days
- These larvae now migrate to mouth parts of black fly. From here they may be transmitted to humans by bite of vector and cycle is repeated
- A provocative test (mazzoti test) may be done. A single dose of 50 mg diethylcarbamazine is administered orally to the patient. The pruritis and rash appearance within 24 hours suggests the presence of microfilariae
- Serological tests like more specific enzyme immunosys using recombinant *Onchocerca volvulus* antigens OC 3.6 and OC 9.3 have been suggested to diagnose onchocerciasis
- Microfilaria antigens in skin samples may be demonstrated by using polymerase chain reactions.

Pathogenicity

- Adult worms develop in subcutaneous tissue after encapsulated in fibrous nodules measuring 5–25 mm. These nodules tend to be present over site where bone is superficial, e.g. hips, knee, iliac crest, ribs, elbow, scalp, coccyx, sacrum, etc.
- Microfilaria may remain localized to site of infection
- Microfilaria may migrate through the adjacent skin to reach tissue, e.g. eyes. In eyes they may result to corneal and retinal lesions leading to blindness. Because of association of black fly with river the disease may be named as River blindness.

Clinical Features

- The disease is called onchocerciasis
- Itching and scratching with secondary infection sometime severe dermatitis occurs called sowda
- Loss of elastic fibers in the skin cause what is known as hanging gown. Actually it is loose hanging containing enlarged lymph node around groin
- There may appear subcutaneous tender nodules
- They are common in the eye with direct spread from adjacent skin appearing to remain mode of spread. Other routes into the eye may be by blood stream along the sheath of posterior ciliary vessels and probably the cerebrospinal fluid along the optic sheath[12]
- Keratitis, irridiocylclitis, optical atrophy and blindness may occur
- The skin wrinkles prematurely, become loose redundant and hypo- or hyperpigmented (leoppart skin).

Laboratory Diagnosis

- Demonstration of adult worm in biopsy
- Demonstration of microfilariae by snipping a small piece of skin with the help of corneal scleral punch or needle and scalpel. The piece of this skin is placed in a drop of normal

saline for 2–4 hours. Microfilariae if present in skin snip can be demonstrated under microscope
- A polymerase chain reaction technique with high specificity for onchocerca volvulus DNA has been developed[13]
- DNA probes are being tested. They can differentiate blinding and non blinding form of onchocercosis.

Treatment

- Surgical removal of detectable nodule can be undertaken
- Ivermectin given orally in a single dose of 150 mg/kg body weight yearly or semiannually is quite effective against microfilaria. It is contraindicated in pregnancy, breastfeeding, CNS disorders and children below 5 years
- DEC can be used in non-ocular onchocerciasis
- Suramin is potentially toxic drug which is capable of killing adult worm. It has no effect on microfilaria.

Prevention and Control

- Applications of insecticides to streams where vector simulium is prevailing. For this DDT or abate may be used
- Because of severe reactions and side effects mass chemotherapy is not recommended
- One must use other physical measures to avoid black fly bites.

REFERENCES

1. Dreyer G, Ottesen EA, Gladino E, et al. Renal abnormalities in microfilariamic patients with Bancroftian filariasis. Am J Trop Med Hyg. 1992;46:745-51.
2. Wucherer OE. Noticia prelimnar sobre vermes de una especic ainda nao descripta encontradosna urina dedoentes de hematuria intrapical bo Brazil. Gaz Med Babia, 1898;3:97–99.
3. Weil GJ, Hussain R, Kumaraswami V, et al. Prenatal allergic sensitization in helminth antigens in offsprings of parasitic infected mothers. J Cl Invest. 1983;71:1124–29.
4. Mc Mahon, JE Marshall, TFC, Vaughan, JP and Abaru DE. Bancroftian filariasis, a comparison of microfilariae counting techniques using counting chamber, standard slide and membrane (nuclepore) filtration. Am Trop Med Parasitol. 1979;73:457-64.
5. Dickerson, JW Eberhard, ML, Lammic PJ. A technique for microfilarial detect in presence of blood using nuclepore filters. J Parasitol. 1990;76:829–33.
6. Rao UR, Lowrie RC, Vickery AC, Kwa B, Nayar JK. A direct fluoscene techniques for the rapid detection of sheathed microfilariae in blood smears. Int J Parasitol. 1990;20:1099-1103.
7. Long GW, Rickman LS, Cross JH. Rapid diagnosis of *Brugia malayi* and *Wuchereria bancrofti* filariasis by an acridine orange microhematolcrittube technique. J Parasitol. 1990;76:278–81.
8. Weiss N, Hussain R, Ottesen E.A. IgE antibodies are more species specific than IgG antibodies in human onchocerciasis and lymphatic filariasis Immunology 1982;45:129-37.
9. Kwan lim G, Forsyth KP, Maizels RM. Filarial specific IgG response co-relatos with active *Wuchereria bancrofti* infection. J Immunol. 1990:4298–2305.
10. Weil GJ, Jain DC, Santhanam Setal. Amonolconal antibody based enzyme assay for detecting parasite antigenemia in bancroftian filariasis. J Infect Dis. 1987;156:350–55.
11. Forsyth KP, Spart R, Kazura J, ct al. A monoclonal antibody based immune radiometric assay for detection of circulating antigen in bancroftian filariasis. J Immunol. 1985;134:1173-77.

12. Duke BO, Vincellette J, Morre PJ. Microfilariae in cerebrospinal fluid and neurological complications during treatment for onchocerciasis with diethyl carbamazine Trop Med Parasitol. 1976;27:125–32.
13. Meredith SEO, Lando G, Gbakima AA, Zimmerman PA, Unnasch TB. Onchorcerca volvulus applications of polymerase chain reaction to identification and strain differentiation of the parasite. Exp Parasitol. 1991;173:335–44.
14. Noireau F, Apember JD. Nzoulani A, et al. Clinical manifestations of loiasis in endemic area in Cango. Trop Med Parasitol. 1990;41:37–39.
15. Klion AD, Massougbodji M, Scadeler BC, et al. Loiasis in endemic and non endemic population: immunological mediated differences in clinical presentation. J Infect Dis. 1991;163:1318–25.
16. Evans TG. Socioeconomic. Consequeneos of blinding oncocerchiasis in West Africa. Bull World Health Organ. 1995;73:495–506.

Oncogenic Helminths

8

INTRODUCTION

Certain helminths possess oncogenic potential and are linked with oncogenesis. Regions of the world endemic for such helminthic infections experience high prevalence of associated cancerous conditions. It is estimated that over 15% malignancies worldwide can be attributed to infections including helminthic infections. Early diagnosis, prompt treatment and prevention of such infections may help in significant reduction in occurrence of these cancerous conditions.[1]

Helminths associated with cancer

I. Blood flukes (Schistosomes): *Schistosoma haematobium*, *Schistosoma mansoni*, *Schistosoma japonicum*

II. Liver flukes: *Opisthorchis viverrini*, *Clonorchis sinensis*, *Opisthorchis felineus*

III. *Taenia solium*: Association of above mentioned helminths with carcinogenesis is discussed as under:

- *Schistosoma haematobium* and *Opisthorchis viverrini* have been found to be strongly associated with bladder cancer and cholangiocarcinoma respectively[1]
- There is ample evidence that *Clonorchis sinensis* is also associated with cholangiocarcinoma[2]
- The evidence for the association of several other parasites and cancers has also been postulated.[1]

SCHISTOSOMIASIS

Schistosomiasis or bilharziasis, caused by infection with trematode *schistosoma* species, is one of the most debilitating helminthic diseases among rural populations, particularly in Sub-Saharan Africa.[3]

There are three major species which affect humans, of which two are predominant in Africa (*Schistosoma haematobium* and *Schistosoma mansoni*) and one is only found in the Far East, mostly in China and Philippines (*Schistosoma japonicum*).[3]

Habitat

- The adult worms of *Schistosoma japonicum* and *Schistosoma mansoni* inhabit the mesenteric veins draining ileo-caecal and sigmoidorectal regions respectively whereas *Schistosoma haematobium* lives primarily in the veins of vesical and pelvis plexuses[4]

- The eggs are deposited in the venules and make their way into the urine or feces.[4]

Pathogenesis

- The immunopathology is due to granuloma formation around the eggs deposited in the tissues and is a manifestation of delayed hypersensitivity reaction, orchestrated by CD4+ T lymphocytes[3,5]
- Large granulomas and fibrosis cause the major pathologic lesions in chronic schistosomiasis.[5]

Association with Cancer

Schistosoma haematobium

- *Schistosoma haematobium* infection is considered a definitive cause of urinary bladder cancer with an associated 5-fold risk[6]
- Bladder cancer is the most prevalent cancer in Egyptians[2]
- Bladder cancer associated with *Schistosoma haematobium* is histologically and pathologically distinct from non *Schistosoma haematobium* associated bladder cancer, the former being a squamous cell carcinoma, with an earlier age of onset and generally sparing the trigone of bladder while the latter is of transitional cell type occurring in the older age group.[1]

Several mechanisms have been suggested to explain the suspected role of *Schistosoma hematobium* in bladder cancer:

- Fibrosis induced by schistosome eggs may induce proliferation, hyperplasia and metaplasia, all of which are possible precancerous changes[7]
- Chronic urinary bacterial infection and production of nitrosamine from their precursors in urine, that are well known bladder carcinogens, from their precursors in urine[8]
- Urinary stasis allowing concentration of endogenous carcinogens leading to their absorption from urine and exposure of the bladder epithelium[9,10]
- Raised urinary beta-glucuronidase levels originating from miracidia and adult schistosomes liberating carcinogenic amines in urine[11]

Schistosoma japonicum

- The evidence supporting role of *Schistosoma japonicum* in cancer occurrence is weaker, although it has been associated with both liver and colorectal cancer[12]
- Thus, presently *Schistosoma japonicum* can be considered a possible carcinogen for humans[1]
- Additional risk factors include viral infection with Hepatitis B (HBV) and Hepatitis C viruses (HCV) and alcohol abuse.[12]

Schistosoma mansoni

- The link between *Schistosoma mansoni* and *Hepatocellular carcinoma* (HCC) appears to be an indirect one[1]
- Patients with *Schistosoma mansoni* have higher rates of HBV and HCV infection compared to non-infected controls, which could be explained partly, by transmission of viruses during parenteral therapy for schistosomiasis.[13,14]
- As cell mediated response is depressed in active intestinal schistosomiasis, these patients tend to retain HBV and HCV for longer periods and attain carrier state with a higher risk of developing complications including Hepatocellular carcinoma.[13]

LIVER FLUKE INFECTIONS

- The human liver flukes *Clonorchis sinensis, Opisthorchis viverrini* and *Opisthorchis felineus,* remain important public health problems in many endemic areas where they infect atleast 20 million people[15]
- *Clonorchis sinensis* is endemic in China, Taiwan, Korea, Japan, and Vietnam; Opisthorchis viverrini is found in Laos and Thailand; Opisthorchis felineus is found in parts of eastern Europe and the former USSR.[16]

Association of liver flukes with cancer

- The most important complication of liver fluke infection is an enhanced susceptibility to cholangiocarcinoma[15]
- *Opisthorchis viverrini* is regarded as a definite human carcinogen causing cholangiocarcinoma whereas evidence for the carcinogenic effect of *Opisthorchis felineus* and *Clonorchis sinensis* is more limited[17]
- However, there is ample evidence that *Clonorchis sinensis* is also associated with cholangiocarcinoma. In Pusan, an area with extremely high prevalence of *C. sinensis,* the fluke increased the risk of cholangiocarcinoma sixfold[18]
- Apart from cholangiocarcinoma, *Opisthorchis viverrini* and *Clonorchis sinensis* have also been linked to hepatocellular carcinoma[1]
- Cases of both cholangiocarcinoma and hepatocellular carcinoma have been reported in people infected with *O. felineus.*[1]

The following possible mechanisms of carcinogenesis due to liver fluke infections have been postulated:

1. **Hyperplasia of bile duct epithelium and carcinogen exposure**: Chronic irritation and chronic inflammation caused by the fluke results in hyperplasia and adenomatous changes of bile duct epithelium. These hyperplastic cells are vulnerable to carcinogens[19]
2. **Increased production of nitric oxide**. In these infections, there is elevated production of nitric oxide in cells. Nitric oxide could have potential genotoxic effects on host by three mechanisms. These include formation of carcinogenic N-nitroso compounds, direct deamination of DNA bases, and oxidation of DNA after formation of peroxynitrite and/or hydroxyl radicals[20]
3. **Increased formation of endogenous carcinogen**: Bile duct epithelial cells are exposed continuously to high concentrations of nitroso compounds being formed in the area of chronic inflammation, leading to neoplastic transformation[21]
4. **Activation of drug metabolizing enzymes**: N-nitrosodimethylamine, one of the products of endogenous nitrosation formed in the tissue, is significantly metabolized by hepatic cytochrome P-450, whose activity is enchanced by *Opisthorchis viverrini* infection. The product of this metabolism is a DNA methylating agent that can result in DNA damage[21]
5. **Aberrant hypermethylation of CpG islands**: CpG islands are often located around the promoters of housekeeping genes. At these locations, the CpG sequence is not methylated in the normal state. Aberrant hypermethylation of CpG islands is a common event observed in liver fluke-related cholangiocarcinogenesis and may potentially contribute to cholangiocarcinogenesis.[22]

NEUROCYSTICERCOSIS

- Produced by cysticerci of the helminth *Taenia solium*[4]
- Develop in man by ingestion of eggs with contaminated water and food or by autoinfection.[4]

Association with Cancer

- Neurocysticercosis has been associated with the emergence of brain tumors particularly glioblastoma multiformae[1]
  Pathogenetic mechanisms explaining possible oncogenic effects of cysticerci include:
  - Chronic inflammation leading to release of nitric oxide in brain which is a potential carcinogen[23]
  - Parasite-induced modulation of the host immune response that may be associated with loss of regulatory mechanisms implicated in the immunological surveillance against cancer[23]
  - Transfer of genetic material from the parasite to the host, causing DNA damage thus predisposing to carcinogenesis[24]
- Neurocysticercosis has also been associated with hematological malignancies[25]
- The chromosomal aberrations induced in peripheral lymphocytes during NCC could be an important factor for association with haematological malignancies.[25]

REFERENCES

1. Khurana S, Dubey ML, Malla N. Association of Parasitic Infections and Cancers. Indian Journal of Medical Microbiology 2005;23(2):74–79.
2. Garcia LS and Bruckner DA. Blood Trematodes. Diagnostic Medical Parasitology, 3rd edn. American Society for Microbiology, Washington DC, ASM Press, 1997:445-77.
3. Fenwick A, Zhang Y. Schistosomiasis. In: Cohen, Powderly, Opal (Eds) Infectious Diseases, 3rd edn, UK: Elsevier; 2010:1171-76.
4. Arora DR, Arora B. Trematodes. Medical Parasitology. 1st edn Reprint. New Delhi,CBS Publishers; 2003:130–51.
5. Maguire JH. Trematodes. In: Mandell, Bennett, Dolin (eds). Principle and Practice of Infectious Diseases, 7th edn. Philadelphia. PA:Churchill Livingstone 2010:3595–605.
6. Pisani P, Parkin DM, Munoz N, Ferlay J. Cancer and infection: Estimates of the artributable fraction in 1990. Cancer Epidemiol Biomarkers Prev. 1997;6:387-400.
7. Rosin MP, Saad El, Din Zaki S, Ward AJ, Anwar WA. Involvement of inflammatory reactions and elevated cell proliferation in the development of bladder cancer in schistosomiasis patients. Mutat Res. 1994;305:283-92.
8. Hicks RM, Ismael MM, Walters CL, et al. Association of bacteriuria and urinary nitrosamine formation with *Schistosoma haematobium* infection in the Qualyub area of Egypt. Trans R Soc Trop Med Hyg. 1982;76:519-28.
9. Bhagwandeen SB. Schistosomiasis and the carcinoma of bladder in Zambia. S Afr Med J 1976;50:1616-20.
10. Cheever AW. Schistosomiasis and neoplasia. J Natl Cancer Inst. 1978;61:13–8.
11. Lucas SB. Squamous cell carcinoma of the bladder and schistosomiasis. East Afr Med J 1982;59:345–51.
12. Ishii A, Matsuoka H, Aji T, Ohta N, Arimoto S, Wataya Y, et al. Parasitic infection and cancer: With special emphasis on Schistosoma japonicum infection (Trematoda). A review. Mutat Res 1994;305:273–81.

13. Lyra LG, Reboucas G, Andrade ZA. Hepatitis B surface antigen carrier state in hepatosplenic schistosomiasis. Gastroenterology 1976;71:641–6.
14. Darwish MA, Raouf TA, Rushdy P. Risk factors associated with a high prevalence of hepatitis C virus infection in Egyptian blood donors. Am J Trop Med Hyg 1993;49:440–9.
15. Haswell-Elkins MR, Elkins DB. Food-Borne Trematodes. In: Gordon Cook, editor. Manson's tropical Diseases. London: WB Saunders; 1996. p. 1458–61.
16. Nash TE. Schistosomiasis and other Trematodes. In: Fauci, Braunwald,Wilson (Eds). Harrisons Principles of Internal Medicine, 14th edn. New York: Mc Graw Hill;1998:1217–23.
17. International agency for Research on cancer. Infection with liver flukes (Opistorchis viverrini, Opisthorrchis felineus and Clonorchis sinensis). IARC Monogr Eval Carcinog Risks Hum 1994;61:121–75.
18. Chung CS, Lee SK. An epidemiological study of primary liver carcinomas in pusan area with special reference to clonorchiasis. Korean J Pathol. 1976;10:33–64.
19. Bhamarapravati N, Thamavit W, Vajrasthira S. Liver changes in hamsters infected with a liver fluke of man, Opisthorchis viverrini. Am J Trop Med Hyg. 1978;27:787–94.
20. Hotchkiss Liu RH,Hotchkiss JH.Potencial genotoxicity of chronically elevated nitric oxide. Mutation Research/Reviews in Genetic Toxicology 1995;339(2):73–83.
21. Kirby GM, Pelkonen P, Vatanasapt V, et. al. Association of liver fluke (*Opistorchis viverrini*) infestation with increased expression of cytochrome P-450 and carcinogen metabolism in male hamster liver. Mol Carcinog 1994;11:81–9.
22. Limpaiboona T, Khaenama P, Chinnasria P. CpG-island methylation study of liver fluke-related cholangoicarcinoma. British Journal of Cancer, 2011;104(8): 1313–18.
23. Del Brutto OH, Dolezal M, Castillo PR, Garcia HH. Neurocysticercosis and oncogenesis. Arch Med Res. 2000;31:151–5.
24. Herrerea LA, Benita A, Sotelo J, et al. Possible relationship between neurocysticercosis and hematological malignancies. Arch Med Res 1999;30:154–8.
25. Herrerea LA, Remirez T, Rodriguez U, et al. Possible association between *Taenia solium* cysticercosis and cancer: Increased frequency of DNA damage in peripheral lymphocytes from neurocysticercosis. Trans R Soc Trop Med Hyg. 2000;94:61–5.

Helminthic Nosocomial Infections

9

Nosocomial infections are also called hospital acquired or hospital associated infections. It is well-known fact that these infections usually complicate 5–10% of all hospitalized patients.[1,2] Nosocomial infections are an important cause of morbidity, mortility and of course increased hospital costs oftenly due to longer stay in the hospital.

Nosocomial in short may be defined as the one diagnosed during or after hospitalization and this particular infection was neither present nor incubating at the time of admission in the hospital. Helminths usually involved in causing infection include *Hymenolepis nana, Taenia solium*, etc. Patient might have acquired the infection many years before hospitalization, e.g. *Strongyloides stercoralis*. The latent infection may get reactivated subsequently when patient becomes debilitated particularly when immune system is suppressed.

Within the hospital complex interaction between food service personal and patients need attention. Food handlers are to be checked closely for harboring helminths. Possible helminthic transmission in healthcare setting is as under:

Table 9.1: Helminths causing nosocomial infections

Helminths	*Mode of transmission*	*Comments*
Enterobius vermicularis	Inhalation and ingestion of infective eggs	Children are involved mostly
Strongyloides stercoralis	Skin penetration of infective larvae from fecal material	Common in immunocompromised patients
Hymenolepis nana	Ingestion of infective eggs (Feco-oral route)	Could cause infection with adult worm in humans
Taenia solium	Ingestion of infective eggs	Could cause cysticercosis

HELMINTHIC GASTROINTESTINAL NOSOCOMIAL INFECTIONS

Nosocomial gastrointestinal may be defined as a acute infectious gastrointestinal illness acquired by a hospitalized patient, especially unexplained diarrhea for 2 days or onset of infectious diarrhea somewhere in the hospital or medical center setting. Helminths involved in gastrointestinal nosocomial infection are:

1. *Hymenolepis nana*: This parasite can be transmitted by the eggs and it does not require intermediate host to complete its life cycle. It is worth mentioning that eggs passed in the stools are mature and infective for patients as well as healthcare workers.
2. *Taenia solium*: An individual harboring adult worm and passing eggs may serve as potential reservoir for transmission of infection. The eggs liberated by *Taenia solium* and passed in stools are mature and infective for both patients and health workers. One must keep in mind the fact that proglottides even kept in preservative contain eggs within uterine branches stay viable and are certainly infective.

NOSOCOMIAL INFECTIONS IN THE IMMUNOCOMPROMISED PERSONS

Immunocompromised persons have poor host defenses may be because of following possibities:

1. Immunosuppression disease (humoral, cellular or both)
2. Chemotherapy or radiations.

Hospital based procedures, e.g. catheterization, nebulizer inhalation procedure, etc.

Contact with infected persons through person-to-person contact, food sources or contaminated equipments and so on *Strongyloides stercoralis* may cause severe disease in immunocompromised patient and may be transmitted in hospital setting. It has become quite important especially in immuno compromised patients,[3] military personal and travellers who have been in an area of endemic infection many years before.[4] Of course persistent undiagnosed disease can be found in these persons. If these persons become immunocompromised the result can be disseminated disease resulting to hyperinfection syndrome and death.[5,6]

A debilitated or compromised patients should always be suspected of having stronglyloidiasis especially if associated with unexplained bouts of diarrhea abdominal pain, repeated sepsis and or meningitis. There is a word of caution for the patients likely to receive immunosuppressive drugs. They must be screened for strongyloidiasis before initiating therapy. If positive for this parasite must be treated properly.

REFERENCES

1. Barrett Connor, ESL, Brandt, JJ Simon, Dechairo DC. Epidemiology for the infection control nurse. The CV Mosby Co., St. Louis, Mo. 1978.
2. Yanelli B, Gurevich PE, Schoch BA, Cunhu. Yield of stool cultures, ova and parasite tests and clostridium difficile determination in nosocomial diarrhoeas. Am J Infect Control. 1988:16:246–49.
3. Jones, CA. clinical studies in human strongyloidiasis. Gastroentrerology 1950; 16:743–56.
4. Pelletier LL Jr. Chronic strongyloidiasis in World War II Far Eat ex prisioner of war. Am J Trop Med Hyg. 1984;33:55–61.
5. Genta RM. Global prevalence of stronglyloidiasis; critical review with epidemiologic insight into the prevention of disseminated disease. Rev Infect Dis 1989;11:755–67.
6. Tabacof J, O Feher, A Katz, SD Simmon and RC Gansi. Strongyloides hyperinfection in two patients with lymphoma, purulent meningitis, and sepsis. Cancer 1991;68:1821–23.

Emerging Helminthic Infections

10

The reasons for emergence of helminthic diseases are:

- Frequent travelling leads to emergence of infectious diseases due to several unique behavioral factors of travellers including:
  - The exotic eating habits abroad and a willingness to eat unfamiliar cuisine raw or undercooked
  - A relaxing of sanitary habits practiced at home, especially frequent handwashing
  - Unfamiliarity with local zoonotic reservoirs of infectious diseases
  - A preference for wilderness, tropical island, and isolated beach resorts that are also home to rodent and other zoonotic reservoir hosts of helminthes.[1]

Overall increase in the number of owning less traditional pets-birds, fish, ferrets, rabbits, and reptiles). This has also led to sudden appearance of helminthic diseases.

The rare but emerging helminthic infections are:

GNATHOSTOMIASIS

Causal Agent

- Gnathostomiasis is a foodborne zoonotic disease caused by several species of the nematode *Gnathostoma*.
- The genus *Gnathostoma* belongs to the order Spirurida, one of the largest groups of nematodes
- In humans: *G. spinigerum, G. hispidum, G. binucleatum* have been reported.[2]

Geographical Distribution

- First discovered in the stomach wall of a tiger that died at London Zoo in 1836 and was first described in humans in 1889 in Thailand by GMR Levinson[2]
- Initially endemic in Japan and Southeast Asia, particularly Thailand, also endemic in Cambodia, Laos, Myanmar, Indonesia, Philippines, and Malaysia, China, Sri Lanka, and India.
- The disease has recently emerged in Mexico, previous reports had identified *G. spinigerum* as the aetiologic agent of gnathostomiasis in Mexico, recent evidence suggests case due to *Gnathostoma binucleatum*.[3]

Reasons for Emergence

Changes in dietary habits due to the consumption of ceviche (raw fish marinated in lime) in Central and South America.[4]

Clinical Features

- Within 24±48 hours of ingestion of *Gnathostoma* spp., patients may develop non-specific signs and symptoms such as malaise, fever, urticaria, anorexia, nausea, vomiting, diarrhea, and epigastric pain.
- Eosinophilia (usually 50%) develops in association with larval penetration of the gastric or intestinal wall.
- The worm migrates through the skin and subcutaneous tissues, causing intermittent swelling that is often painful or pruritic.
- The worm can migrate to deeper tissues, resulting in visceral disease and involve the pulmonary, ocular, genitourinary, gastrointestinal, auditory, and central nervous systems, occasionally with fatal consequences.[4]

Treatment

Definitive cure of gnathostomiasis can be achieved by :
- Extraction of the infective larvae from the subcutaneous tissues.
- With albendazole therapy, patients can be cured medically.[4]

Prevention

Rather, control of gnathostomiasis will only be achieved through intensive education campaigns to raise public awareness of this foodborne helminthic zoonosis.[4]

ESOPHAGOSTOMIASIS

Causal Agent

Oesophagostomum bifurcum, the parasite is a member of the hookworm family of strongylid parasites, and is a common intestinal nematode of primates.[5]

Geographical Distribution

- Human infection with the nematode parasite *Oesophagostomum bifurcum*, was until recently considered a rare zoonosis. In 1991 Polderman, et al. reported that the parasite was commonly found in humans in Northern Togo and Ghana
- Recent estimates indicate that in these areas over 230,000 individuals carry infection.[6]

Clinical Features

- The most prominent clinical manifestation of infection is the so-called `Dapaong tumor', named after the capital of Togo's northernmost fsprovince, an inflammatory mass around juvenile worms, either within the colonic wall or in the abdominal cavity
- The presence of pain is variable, and secondary complications such as colonic obstruction may occur
- Rare manifestations include ectopic disease in the omentum, liver or skin.[7]

Treatment

The infection is responsive to albendazole and pyrantel palmoate.[7]

CAPILLARIASIS

Causal Agent

- Although more than 250 species of *Capillaria* have been identified, only three are known to infect humans: *Capillaria philippinensis, Capillaria hepatica*, and *Capillaria aerophilia.*
- Of the three, *C. philippinensis* is the only species of significance, and potentially an emerging zoonotic helminth.[8]

Geographical Distribution

- *C. philippinensis* infection was first described in rural communities in the Philippines in 1965
- However, the geographic extent of infection has continued to widen, with cases recorded in Indonesia, Japan, Taiwan, India, Iran, and Egypt. This zoonotic nematode parasite has emerged in the past 20 years.[8]

Reasons for Emergence

The parasite is enzootic in sheating birds. The fish contract infection from the feces of infected birds, or from fecal contamination of water by infected humans. Humans become infected by eating uncooked small fresh water fish.[9]

Clinical Features

- Leads to progressive small bowel dysfunction, marked by diarrhea, abdominal pain, malabsorption and weight loss
- Infection is frequently fatal in the absence of appropriate anthelmintic chemotherapy.[9]

Treatment

- Albendazole, given in a dose of 200 mg twice daily for 10 days is the preferred treatment.
- Mebendazole, in a dose of 100 mg twice daily is an acceptable alternative, but needs to be given for 20 days, and relapses are more frequent with this drug.[9]

ANISAKIDOSIS

Causal Agent: Anisakis simplex, a nematodal infection.

Geographical Distribution

The greatest experience of anisakidosis is in Japan, where the consumption of raw fish has been a standard cultural practice for centurie, the annual incidence was reported to exceed 2000 cases in Japan alone.[10]

Reasons for Emergence

Two factors have been cited to explain the rise of anisakidosis as an emerging parasitic disease, one dietary (due to comsumption of raw fish), and the other environmental.[11]

Clinical Features

- It may be dominated by allergic response. Sensitisation may result in urticaria, angioedema or anaphylaxis after eating infected seafood, the local allergic response result in intestinal obstruction, and mesenteric adenitis mimicking the symptoms of appendicitis.
- This syndrome may be responsible for a significant proportion of cases of so-called idiopathic eosinophilic gastroenteritis.[12]

Treatment

- Endoscopic removal of the larva is curative.[12]

EOSINOPHILIC ENTERITIS (*ANCYLOSTOMA CANINUM*)

Causal Agent

- It is caused by Ancylostoma caninum, parasites of dogs and are capable of producing the larva migrans syndromes in humans, causes eosinophilic enteritis
- In the US, this condition is mainly due to Ancylostoma braziliensis, a parasite that is common in both dogs and cats.[13]

Geographical Distribution

A. caninum has an almost worldwide distribution, *A. caninum*-induced eosinophilic enteritis infection is endemic in Australia. Isolated case reports due to *A. caninum* in South America, the Philippines, Israel and the US.[13]

Reasons for Emergence

The number of infected individuals has expanded greatly as a result of two factors, namely the increased awareness of the entity, and the high prevalence of dog ownership.[14]

Clinical Features

Cutaneous larva migrans is characterised by progressive linear eruptive lesions due to the prolonged subcutaneous migration of this zoonotic hookworm larvae.[14]

Treatment

Albendazole is efficacious.

Prevention

An effective surveillance and control program would necessitate attention to potentially infected dogs.[14]

BAYLISASCARISIS

Causal Agent

Baylisascaris procyonis, a roundworm infection of raccoons, is emerging as an important helminthic zoonosis, principally affecting young children.[15]

Geographical Distribution

Baylisascaris procyonis has been identified in the United States, Europe, and Japan, South America.[15]

Reasons for Emergence

Baylisascaris procyonis is thought to pose the greatest risk to humans because of the often close association of raccoons to human dwellings.[15]

Clinical features

- Skin irritations from larvae migrating within the skin.
- Respiratory discomfort, liver enlargement, and fever due to reaction to larvae migration.
- Eye and brain tissue damage due to the random migration of the larvae.
- Nausea, a lethargic feeling, incoordination and loss of eyesight.
- Severe neurological signs caused by extensive tissue damage due to larval migration through the brain, eventually seizures and coma.[16]

Treatment

No treatment has been shown to alleviate illness caused by migrating larvae. Despite lack of larvicidal effects, albendazole (20–40 mg/kg/d for 1–4 weeks) has been used to treat many cases.

Prevention

- Discouraging raccoon access to home sites and neighborhoods
- Discouraging keeping raccoons as domestic pets or importing raccoons as exotic pets;
- Recognizing that infective eggs are environmentally stable and resistant to common household disinfectants including ammonia, bleach, and chlorhexidine and can only be removed from the hands by vigorous soap and water washing and not simply by hand sanitizers
- Controlling raccoon populations in residential areas with trapping and relocation programs.[16]

ANGIOSTRONGYLIASIS

Causal Agents

The nematode (roundworm) *Angiostrongylus cantonensis*, the rat lungworm—most common cause of human eosinophilic meningitis. Angiostrongylus (Parastrongylus) costaricensis—the causal agent of abdominal, intestinal angiostrongyliasis.[16]

The Epidemiology of Neuroangiostrongyliasis

- Neuroangiostrongyliasis, a rodent zoonosis, is now endemic in the United States (US) following the introduction of giant African land snails as biological controls and exotic pets. *A. cantonensis* is the most common infectious cause of EM in humans in the US and worldwide.
- Enzootic throughout Southeast Asia, most Indian and Pacific Ocean islands.[16]

Reason for Emergence

- The rapid global spread of the parasite resulted from infected rat on container ships docked at port cities
- The intentional introduction of giant African land snails, as biological controls for commercial agricultural operations and as exotic pets for home terrariums.
- The lettuce food contaminated somewhere with snails or slugs or their secretions also contains infective *A. cantonensis* larvae and is presumed to be reason for emergence.[17]

Clinical Features

- After incubation period of approximately 2 weeks, patients with NAS will typically present as aseptic meningitis with headache, stiff neck, nausea, vomiting, low-grade to no fever (especially in adults), and asymmetrical hyperesthesias or paresthesias in the extremities that are frequently overlooked
- Papilledema and transient cranial nerve palsies, most commonly facial nerve palsies, may occur
- Permanent neurologic sequelae and death are rare, and most patients recover completely within 2 weeks.[17]

Treatment

- Since most cases of NAS resolve spontaneously, treatment is often supportive and nonspecific.[1] The anthelminthics, albendazole and praziquantel, are effective larvicides
- Adjunctive corticosteroids may ameliorate this inflammatory response.[17]

Prevention

Effective prevention and control strategies for NAS include the following:

- Educating citizens and travelers in endemic areas that snails, slugs, freshwater fish and shrimp, frogs, and crabs must be cooked thoroughly, not simply marinated or refrigerated before being eaten;
- Washing all fruits and vegetables before eating them uncooked;
- Reducing and controlling the definitive host rodent populations with rodenticides;
- Reducing and controlling snail with molluscicides.[17]

REFERENCES

1. Ryan ET, Wilson ME, Kain KC. Illness after international travel. N Engl J Med. 2002;347:505–16.
2. Boongird P, Phuapradit P, Siridej N, Chirachariyavej T, Chuahirun S, Vejjajiva A. Neurological manifestations of gnathostomiasis J Neurol Sci 1977;31:279–91.
3. Rusnak JM, Lucey DR. Clinical gnathostomiasis: case report and review of the English-language literature. Clin Infect Dis. 1993;16:33–50.
4. Nawa Y, C Hatz, and J Blum. 22 Sushi delights and parasites: the risk of fishborne and foodborne parasitic zoonoses in Asia. Clin Infect Dis. 2005;41:1297–1303.
5. McCarthy J, Moore TA. Emerging helminth zoonoses. Int J Parasitol. 2000;1351-60.
6. Polderman AM, Krepel HP, Baeta S, et al. Oesophagostomiasis, a common infection of man in Northern Togo and Ghana. Am J Trop Med Hyg. 1991;44:336–44.
7. Storey PA, Anemana S, van Oostayen JA, et al. Ultrasound diagnosis of oesophagostomiasis. Br J Radiol. 2000;73:328–32.

8. Chitwood MB, Vaalasquez C, Salazar NG, et al. The physiological changes in a species of *Capillaria* causing a fatal case of human intestinal capillariasis. Proc First Int Congr Parasitol. 2000.
9. Cross JH. Intestinal capillariasis. Clin Microbiol Rev. 1992;5:120–9.
10. Moreno-Ancillo A, Caballero MT, Cabanas R, et al. Allergic reactions to anisakis simplex parasitizing seafood. Ann Allergy Asthma Immunol. 1997;79:246–50.
11. van Thiel PH, Kuipers FC, Roskam RT. A nematode parasite to herring causing acute abdominal syndromes in man. Trop Geogr Med. 1960;2:97–113.
12. Kagei N, Orikasa H, Hori E, et al. A case of hepatic anisakiasis with a literal survey for extra-intestinal anisakiasis. Jpn J Parasitol. 1995;44:346–51.
13. Prociv P, Croese J. Human eosinophilic enteritis caused by dog hookworm *Ancylostoma caninum*. Lancet 1990;335:1299–302.
14. Walker NI, Croese J, Clouston AD, et al. Eosinophilic enteritis in Northeastern Australia. Pathology, association with *Ancylostoma caninum*, and implications. Am J Surg Pathol. 1995;19:328–37.
15. Park SY, Glaser C, Murray WJ, et al. Raccoon roundworm (*Baylisascaris procyonis*) encephalitis: case report and field investigation. Pediatrics. 2000;106:E56.
16. James H Diaz. Recently Reemerging Helminthic Infections Causing Eosinophilic Meningo-encephalitis: Neuroangiostrongyliasis, Baylisascariasis, and Gnathostomiasis. J Neuroparasitol Vol. 1 2010 Article ID N100503.
17. Cuneo P, Clement S, Sokol T. *Eosinophilic meningitis* and *Angiostrongylus cantonensis*, Louisiana Morbid Rep. 2006;17:1.

Helminthic Control, Preventive Measures and Vaccines

11

CONTROL OF HELMINTHS INFECTIONS

No helminthic has been eradicated although there are serious attempts in this direction. Eradication of Guinea worm is on way with full force, through programme Global 2000. Success has been attained in elimination of Guinea worm in some local areas. Other examples include:

- Onchocercosis has been eliminated from parts of Kenya and from the Nile at Jinja in Uganda by using insecticides dichlodiphenyltrichloroethane (DDT) to remove local vector, i.e. *Simulium neavei* and *Simulium damnosum* respectively
- Onchocercosis in West Africa is eliminated targeting cytoforms of *S. damnosum* complex using insecticides
- Local antmosquito spraying has eliminated lymphatic filariasis from Solomon islands with no resurgence over 20 years time
- *Brugia malayi* filariasis eliminated from Sri Lanka with the use of drug diethylcarbamazine (DEC), antilarval (by removing herbiciding—host plants) measures and environmental improvement
- Use of chemotherapeutics to eliminate filariasis caused by *Wuchereria bancrofti* from Japan, South Korea and Taiwan in Asia and Suriname along with Trinidad and Tobago in America[2]
- Filariasis has been eliminated as public health problem in large area of China.

Preventive Measures to Avoid Helminthic Infections

In real sense prevention of helminthic infection is based on various helminthic life cycle and modes of infection. Preventive measures are usually revolve around personal hygiene and sanitation. Preventive measures include as under:

- It is desirable to avoid ingestion of soil contaminated with helminths eggs, e.g. hookworm, roundworm, etc.
- Adequate cooking of infected meat should be done
- Vector control including protection of well water sources
- Proper treatment of patients harboring helminths, e.g. tapeworms
- Proper attention must be given to personal hygiene and sanitation measures
- It is always required to avoid eating raw water plants that might contain encysted larval forms of the flukes
- Adequate disposal of waste of form animals feces (pigs) especially concerning flukes
- There should be thorough cooking of potentially infected fish, crabs, crayfish, etc. to avoid trematodes (liver lung). They might contain encysted metacercariae
- Protection from potentially contaminated water sources and proper handling of human waste containing eggs (infection of small intermediate host)

- Elimination of sexual activities where there is possibility for fecal oral contact
- Adequate water treatment like filtration must be made available
- Chemoprophylactic agents must be used to patients who plan to travel to endemic areas
- Vector control, blood transfusion, shared drug needles, congenital infections and organ transplant are important aspects to prevent human diseases caused by parasites. Monitoring of blood supply is needed for helminths transmitted via blood.

HELMINTHIC VACCINES

All over the world morbidity due to prevalence of helminths and infection and thereafter resulting into ill health morbidity in human is a reason of concern. This problem does a major impact on socio economic development especially when lack of hygiene poor mutation and iron availability are prevalent around.

HELMINTHIC VACCINE DEVELOPMENT CHALLENGES AND PROBLEMS

- Helminths being multicellular consists of many varieties of cells with different functions. Their elimination raise a challenge as it require unusual mechanism to get rid of them
- They have multiple stages in their life cycle
- In *Trichinella spiralis* and *Brugia* species some antigen may be released in circulation which may act as smoke screen to induce antibodies or immune response
- Helminths many a time may acquire host molecules and so may not be recognized as non-self by immune system. Acquisition of ABO blood group substances may occur by schistosomula of *Schistosoma mansoni*
- Since helminths by and large do not multiply within human host, total burden in man is usually dependent basically on repeated exposure to infectious parasitic forms.

PROTECTIVE HELMINTH ANTIGENS AND EPITOPES

- On the basis of the ability to induce protective immunity in experimental animals
- Selection of candidate protective antigens considering known metabolic functions of the parasitic molecules
- Antigens selected based on lack of detectable immune response to moleculic in natural occurring helminthic infections.

GOALS OF AN IDEAL HELMINTHIC VACCINE

1. To induce resistance to infective larval stages to prevent infection of host.
2. To kills adult stage parasite thus eliminating parasite in previously infected individual.
3. Preparing antipathology vaccine to prevent disease manifestations.
4. To provide resistance to parasitic stages involved in helminthic transmission. This decreases the availability to vector. It may thus interrupt life cycle.
5. To make available transmission blocking immunity which may impair development of helminths in obligate intermediate host.

Immunoglobulin genes can be rearranged and their final protein production may be monitored. Gene rearrangement and slicing techniques can be made useful. Antibodies of many different specificities may be synthesized from a relatively small number of genes for certain purposes. Likewise many helminthic vaccines might be developed.

In future many novel helminthic vaccines may be prepared need of which is now felt more intensely to reduce their incidence and mobility associated with them. Need for having helminthic vaccines is required essentially because of:

1. Drugs do not eradicate infection in the host but impact eliminate only one stage of the helminths. Obviously it warrants periodic treatment.
2. Development of drug resistance in helminths make it less effective.
3. There are always chance of repeated helminthic infections because of prevailing conditions around.
4. Expensive and at the same time repeated drug treatment is becoming beyond tolerance to involved persons.

Vaccines in Helminthic Parasites

The goals of anthelmintic vaccines are different from those of conventional antiviral and antibacterial vaccination. In parasites, it is unlikely that immunization with defined antigens will elicit sterilizing immunity against complex metazoan organisms. So the most important goal that remains is to reduce the worm burden below the disease causing threshold. The essential concept of anthelmintic vaccine is to attempt to immunize against disease rather than infection. For instance, to reduce hookworm burden below the threshold that results in significant intestinal blood loss which leads to anemia or to reduce the schistosome burden below the threshold that results in significant egg deposition and subsequent granuloma formation in liver, intestines and bladder.[3]

Another approach to anti-disease vaccination would be to directly block the action of parasite induced pathogenic processes. In hookworm, this would require blocking parasite derived virulence factors that cause blood loss and in schistosomes for blocking egg deposition.

It will not be possible to use anthelminthic vaccines alone but in conjunction with other control measures including conventional chemotherapy.[4]

Vaccines for Hookworm Disease

Human hookworm infection is the leading cause of anemia and malnutrition among children in developing countries in regions of Sub Saharan Africa, Asia and tropical America.[5,6] *Ancylostoma duodenale* and *Necator americanus* are the major hookworms worldwide. After varying attempts at developing a hookworm vaccine, a class of antigens which looks promising is the Ancylostoma-secreted proteins (ASPs), which are released by host stimulated L3.[7,8] X-irradiated L3 vaccine[9,10] has proved protective against challenge with animal hookworms.[11,12] A reduction in risk of having heavy hookworm infection has also been seen with human anti-ASP2 antibody responses. A pilot study being conducted by the Human Hookworm Vaccine Initiative at the Sabin Vaccine Institute in Washington, DC has developed hookworm vaccine using ASP-2 from *Necator americanus* (Na-ASP-2) expressed in yeast.[13] This vaccine has undergone phase 1 trials for safety and immunogenecity in the United States, using three doses of either 10, 50 or 100 μg given at 0, 4 and 8 weeks and found to be safe and immunogenic. Trails are now being planned in hookworm endemic areas of Brazil.[12]

A second approach to hookworm vaccination makes use of the fact that various proteolytic enzymes line the brush border membrane of hookworm gastrointestinal tract which help the parasite in digesting haemoglobin.[14] Vaccination with a recombinant aspartic hemoglobinase, APR-1 has been shown to reduce parasite load and blood loss following hookworm infection in dogs.[15]

These trials with different antigens will lead to development of a vaccination strategy acting in conjunction with conventional chemotherapy.[8,13]

Vaccines for Schistosomiasis

Schistosomes are water borne, snail transmitted trematodes. The main species of schistosomes are *Schistosoma hematobium, S. mansoni* and *S. japonicum*.

Many different approaches have been tried to develop a vaccine against schistosomal infection. Vaccine antigens from different schistosomal stages have been developed as potential candidate vaccines. But the protection achieved in reducing the worm burden or egg count is less than 40%.

Better protection has been seen with using antigens shared between schistosomula and adult schistosomes which include parasite derived myosin(63kDa), paramyosin(97kDa), triose phosphate isomerase (28kDa), glutathione-S-transferases(GSTs:26 and 28kDa), a fatty acid binding protein(14kDa) and a 23kDa surface protein. Most of these experiments have been conducted in mice challenged with either *S. mansoni* or *S. japonicum*.[16]

Recombinant antigen based vaccine trials have also been conducted using different adjuvants like Fruend's complete adjuvant, alum, Bacille Calmette-Guerin (BCG), saponin, Quil A and Bordetella pertussis.[16]

Another approach to anti-schistosomal vaccine has been to target the fecundity of female adult schistosomes to decrease the egg excretion into target host organs. For this 26kDa and 28kDa variants of glutathione-S-transferase have been tried in mice, non-human primates and large animal reservoir hosts including pigs and water buffaloes.[16,17]

During the late 1990s, WHO's special programme for Research and Training in Tropical Diseases initiated murine trials of six vaccine candidates for *S. mansoni* but all showed less than 40% efficacy.[18]

Recently, a membrane spanning schistosome surface protein (tetraspanin) has been identified that results in 60-70% worm burden reductions in mice.[17] Studies are being done to determine the feasibility for this class of antigen.

The Pasteur Institute in Lille, France has produced a 28kDa GST from *Schistosoma haematobium* (Sh28GST) in yeast under cGMP and conducting clinical trials.[15] Among human volunteers' two subcutaneous injections of 100 µg of recombinant Sh28GST in alum resulted in an immune response comprising predominantly of IgG1 and IgG3.[17] Evaluation of its clinical efficacy and synergy with praziquantel therapy is being conducted.

Vaccines against Teniasis

Taenia solium, the pork tapeworm is a cause of an important human infection, neurocysticercosis. It is potentially eradicable if the transmission from pigs to humans is interrupted. One of the approaches being tried is the use of recombinant oncosphere antigen, two of which, designated TSOL18 and TSOL45 have been evaluated.[20] These have induced complete or near complete protection against experimental challenge infection in vaccine trials in pigs. This vaccine can contribute substantially to control and eradicate human neurocysticercosis.

HUMAN ANTI-HELMINTHIC DISEASE VACCINES UNDER DEVELOPMENT

Table 11.1: Human anti-helminthic disease vaccines under development

Pathogen	*Promising Antigens*	*Status*
Necator americanus (hookworm)	Na ASP-2 (ancylostoma secreted protein)	Phase 1
	Na-APR-1 (aspartic protease)	Preclinical
	Na-GST-1 (glutathione S-transferase)	Preclinical
Echinococcus granulosus (Hydatid disease)	Eg95	Veterinary (transmission blocking)
Onchocerca volvulus (river blindness)	Ov-ASP-1 (ancylostoma secreted protein)	Preclinical
	Ov-7 (onchocystatin)	Preclinical
Schistosoma haematobium	Sh28GST (glutathione S-Transferase)	Phase 2
Schistosoma mansoni	Sm-TSP-2 (tetraspanin)	Preclinical
	Sm-14 (fatty acid binding protein)	
	Sm-23	
	Sm-28 (triose phosphate isomerase)	
	Sm-97 (paramyosin)	
Schistosoma japonicum	Sj-97 (paramyosin)	Veterinary (transmission blocking)
	Sj28GST (glutathione S-transferase)	
	Sj26GST (glutathione S-transferase)	
Taenia solium (cysticercosis)	TSOL18 (onchosphere antigen)	Veterinary (transmission blocking)
	TSOL45-1A (onchosphere antigen)	

Prospects of Helminthic Vaccines

New prospects of emergence of new vaccines are very much in sight. Schistosome and filariasis vaccines are becoming the reality of the day.

With respect to candidate peptide and protein antigens, the problems of laying hand to sufficient quantity of material from limited supply of helminths has been compensated by molecular cloning. Moreover in view of better understanding of role of B and T cell responses and protective immunity, there is definitely the possibility of candidate helminth vaccine in coming future.

REFERENCES

1. Hopkins DR, Withers PC. Sudan's war and eradication of dracunculiasis Lancet, 360, Supplement 2002:521–22.
2. WHO 1994. Lymphatic filariasis and disease control strategies. Report of a consultative meeting Penang, Malaysia Division of control of Tropical Diseases (CTD) and UNDS/World Bank/WHO spread programme for Research and Training in Tropical Diseases (TDR), TDR/CTD/FIL/PENANG. Geneva World Health Organization, 1994.
3. Brooker S, Bethony JM, Rodrigues LC, et al. Epidemiologic, immunologic and practical considerations in developing and evaluating a human hookworm vaccine. Expert Rev Vaccines 2005;4:35–50.
4. Bergquist NR, Leonardo LR, Mitchell GF. Vaccine linked chemotherapy: can schistosomiasis control benefit from an integrated approach. Trends Parasitol 2005;21:112–17.
5. Hotez PJ, Brooker S, Bethony JM, et al. Hookworm infection. N Engl J Med 2004;351:799–807.
6. Bethony J, Brooker S, Albonico M, et al. Soil transmitted helminth infections: ascariasis, trichuriasis and hookworm. Lancet 2006;367:1521–32.
7. Asojo OA, Goud G, Dhar K, et al. X-ray structure of Na-ASP-2, a pathogenesis related 1 protein from the nematode parasite Necator americanus, and a vaccine antigen for human hookworm infection. J Mol Biol. 2005;346:801–04.
8. Hotez PJ, Loukas A, Bottazzi ME, et al. Hookworm:the greatest infection of mankind' PloS Medicine 2005;2:e67.
9. Fujiwara RT, Loukas A, Mendez S, et al. Vaccination with irradiated Ancylostome caninum third stage larvae induce a Th2 response in Dogs. Vaccine 2006;24:501–9.
10. Bethony J, Loukas A, Smout M, et al. Antibodies against a secreted protein from hookworm larvae reduces the intensity of hookworm infection in humans and vaccinated laboratory animals. FASEB J. 2005;19:1743–45.
11. Goud GN, Bottazzi ME, Khan B, et al. Expression of Necator americanus hookworm larval antigen Na-ASP-2 in Pichia pastoris and purification of the recombinant protein for use in human clinical trials. Vaccine 2005;23:4754–64.
12. Goud GN, Khan B, Ghosh K, et al. Cloning, yeast expression, isolation and vaccine testing of recombinant Ancylostoma secreted protein(ASP)-1 and ASP-2 from Ancylostome ceylanicum. J Infect Dis. 2004;189;919–29.
13. Hotez PJ, Bethony J, Bottazzi ME, et al. New technologies fro the control of human hookworm infection. Trends Parasitol. 2006;22; 327–31.
14. Williamson AL, Lecchi B, Turk BE, et al. A multienzyme cascade of heamoglobin proteolysis in the intestine of blood feeding hookworms. J Biol Chem. 2004;279:35950–7.
15. Loukas A, Bethony J, Mendez S, et al. Vaccination with recombinant aspartic hemoglobonase reduces parasite load and blood loss after hookworm infection in dogs. PloS Medicine 2005 2:e295.
16. McManus DP. Prospects for development of a transmission blocking vaccine against Schistisoma japonicum. Parasit Immunol. 2005;27:297–308.
17. Capron A, Riveau G, Capron M, Trottein F.Schistosomes: the road from host parasite interactions to vaccines in clinical trials. Trends Parasitol. 2005;21:143–9.
18. Doenhoff M. A vaccine for schistosomiasis: alternative approaches. Parasitol Today 1998:14;105-9.
19. Tran MH, Pearson MS, Bethony JM, et al. Tetraspanins on the surface of Schistosoma mansoni are protective vaccine antigens in mice and Sm-TSP-2 is selectively recognised by naturally resistant individuals. Nat Med. (Epub ahead of print), 2006.
20. Lightowlers MW. Vaccines against cysticercosis and hydatidosis: Foundations in taeniid cestode immunology. Parasitol Int. 2006;55 Suppl: S39-S43.

12 Treatment of Intestinal Helminthiasis

1. Specific diagnosis should be established before planning treatment. Multiple helminthic infections quite common especially in tropical countries. One needs to decide specific therapy to helminthic diseases causing serious and greater pathogenic effects.
2. Patients suffering from helminthic problems must be examined and assessed carefully especially regarding anemia, cirrhosis of liver, nephritis and pregnancy. Almost majority of anthelminthic drugs are not tolerated by alcoholics. For this reason consumption of alcohol should be stopped by patients.
3. It is a must that worms are exposed to direct action of drugs. For this light diet in the evening and sometimes a purgative at night before administering anthelminthic drugs should be given.
4. Antehelminthic may be administrated in the morning on an empty stomach.
5. No edible to be given upto 2 hours after specific medication.
6. Sometime post-purgative is obligatory to expel the injured parasites which might recover if left in the intestine. If the parasite are disintegrated it may release toxic material giving rise to toxic manifestations. Further post-purgative may prevent any absorption of drug which may reduce drug toxicity.
7. Food is permitted till bowel move.
8. All stool samples should be collected and examined for the worms expelled.
9. It is advised to carry on follow-up examination of stool to evaluate the success of treatment. Second course of treatment have to be repeated if there is evidence of presence of helminthics.

AGENTS USED IN HELMINTHIC DISEASES

Helminthic diseases impose substantial health problems in global developing nations where they are more prevalent. We have been successful in checking or eradication some of these conditions like dracunculiasis, onchocerciasis and so on. Some helminthic conditions have extensively expanded because of deforestation, population shifts, global warming and other climatic mishappenings. It is a hard fact that chemotherapy remains only effective way of checking helminthic problems. On the other front, we have engaged with development of vaccine too. Chemotherapy has limitations because of emergence of drug resistance and practically non addition of newer anthelminthic agents. Expensive agents like praziquantel and metrifonate is being diffident to prescribe to poor patients.

Albendazole and ivermection has contributed significally towards eradication programmes and improving the health of countless persons. Hopefully, we are going toward eradication of some problems, e.g. filariasis. Some anthelminthic drugs are discussed as under:

ALBENDAZOLE (ZENTEL, ALMINTH, ALBEZOLE)

It acts by binding free B tubulin, inhibiting the polymerization of tubulin and microtubulin dependent uptake of glucose. Basically there is disruption of cellular metabolism. Albendazole is poorly absorbed from gastrointestinal tract which is infact useful in helminthic diseases.

In helminthic diseases, e.g. hydatid or neurocysticercosis, sufficient quantity active drug must reach the site of infection. Actually metabolite albendazole sulfoxide is responsible for curative effect outside the gut lumen. As such significant quantum of this metabolite is found in lungs, liver tissue and hydatid fluid.

Albendazole sulfoxide does cross blood brain barrier, a level quite higher than attained in plasma. The higher level of albendazole sulfoxide in cerebrospinal fluid (CSF) explain the efficacy of albendazole in the treatment of neurocysticercosis.

A single dose of 400 mg is generally recommended to treat gastrointestinal nematode. This dose is largely without any side effects. When administrated for long period (e.g. cystic and alveolar hydrated disease) may be associated with abnormal liver function and bone marrow toxicity. In such situations, albendazole may be given in cycles of 28 days interrupting by 14 days off treatment.

It is administered orally and it attains peak plasma concentration in about 2 hours. The drug is mostly eliminated by kidney excretion. Alkalization of urine enhances half-life of drug by decreasing excretion of drug. No parenteral form of this drug is available.

Adverse Effect

There may be dose related nausea, vomiting. Patient may develop rarely fever, chills, arthralgia and headache.

IVERMECTIN (IVERMECTOL, IVERMEC, VERMIN)

It is a derivative of the macrocylic lactone avermectin produced by *Streptomyces avermitilis* (soil *Actinomyces*). It is a drug of choice to treat onchocerciasis, strongyloidiasis, cutaneous larva migrans, etc. It is worth mentioning that this drug is highly active against microfilaria of lymphatic filariasis. It is active against intestinal helminthiasis especially ascariasis and entrobiasis. It is partially effective against trichuriasis. It is not effective against hookworm.

Ivermectin is available as only oral preparation because of its low water solubility. The dose recommended is 150–200 μg/kg body weight.

Indications

- Ascariasis
- Cutaneous larva migrans
- Entrobiasis
- Loiasis
- Lymphatic filariasis
- Onchocerciasis
- Strongyloidiasis
- Ascariasis
- Clonorchiasis
- Cysticercosis

- Echinococcosis
- Hookworm infection
- Trichinellosis
- Trichuriasis
- Visceral larva migrans.

Side Effects

- Nausea
- Vomiting
- Abdominal pain
- Headache
- Reversible alopecia
- Elevated aminotransferases
- Rarely leukopenia and rash.

Drug Interactions

- Dexamethasone
- Praziquantel.

DIETHYLCARBAMAZINE (HETRAZAN, BANOCIDE)

It remains the drug of choice for lymphatic filariasis, loasis and visceral larva migrans. It causes immobilization of worms due to decreased muscle activity, etc., resulting in enhanced killing by host's immune system. It also enhances adherence feature of eosinophils. This drug may be given monthly to have prophylactic benefit of bancroftian filariasis and loiasis.

Side Effects

- Fever
- Pruritis
- Headache
- Myalgia
- Rarely hypotension.

Contraindications

- Pregnancy
- Excreted in breast milk.

MEBENDAZOLE

It is a broad spectrum antiparasitic agent used against intestinal helmenthiasis. It is available only in oral form. It is poorly absorbed from gastrointestinal tract and so low incidence of side effects. Rare and temporary side effects include abdominal pain and diarrhea which occur in patient with heavy parasitic burden.

Indications

- Ascariasis
- Entrobiasis
- Hookworm
- Trichinellosis
- Trichostrongylidiasis
- Trichuriasis
- Visceral larva migrans.

Side Effects

- Diarrhea
- Abdominal pain
- Elevated aminotransferases
- Rarely agranulocytosis, thrombocytopenia and alopecia.

Drug Interaction

- Cimetidine inhibits mebendazole metabolism.

Contraindication

- Pregnancy.

METRIFONATE

It is active against *Schistosoma hematobium*. It is believed to exert its effect by virtue of inhibiting tegumental acetylecholine receptors that mediate glucose transport. Otherwise its mechanism of action remains uncertain.

It is administered in series of three doses at 2 weeks intervals. Treated persons may not be exposed to neuromuscular blocking agents or organophosphate compounds for at least 48 hours after treatment.

Indications

- Schistosomiasis.

Side Effect

- Frequent abdominal pain
- Nausea
- Vomiting
- Diarrhea
- Headache
- Vertigo
- Bronchospasm.

NICLOSAMIDE

It is effective against adult tapeworm. However it is not useful against tissue cestode. It action is to inhibit oxidative phosphorylation of mitochondria of worm ultimately resulting to deprivation of energy.

It is poorly absorbed and administered empty stomach in the morning after a liquid meal the night before. It is followed by another dose of drug after a lapse of 1 hour. For Hymenolepiasis drug may be administered for 7 days and it may require second course of treatment. On coming into contact of drug with scolex and proximal segment of tapeworm may get killed. At the same time it may cause disintegration and digestion of tapeworm. It results to releasing of viable ova and thus leading to autoinfection. It is suggestive that brisk purgative must be given two hours after the first dose of niclosamide.

Indications

- Intestinal cestodes.

Side Effects

- Nausea
- Vomiting
- Dizziness
- Pruritis.

OXAMNIGUINE

Useful to treat *Schistosoma mansoni* infections. It exerts anticholinergic effect although primary mode of its effect is on ATP dependent enzymatic drug activation generating an intermediate that alkylates essential macromolecules including DNA. Oxaminoquine may cause tegumental alteration taking 4–8 days after treatment.

It is given orally as a single dose. However food slows absorption of drug and bioavailability. It is excreted through urine giving intense orange red color to urine. This drug may cause hallucinations and seizures as side effects.

Indications

- Schistosomiasis.

Side Effects

- Dizziness
- Drowsiness
- Headache
- Orange colored urine
- Elevated aminotransferases
- Seizures.

PRAZIQUANTEL (CYSTICIDE, DISTOCIDE)

It is highly active against trematodes and cestodes. It remains main treatment of schistosomiasis and is considered vital part of community based control programme.

Praziquantel induces changes in antigenicity of the parasites by exposing hidden antigens. It also causes alteration of schistosomal glucose metabolism which decreases in glucose intake, lactate release, glycogen contents and ATP levels. There is disruption of the parasitic tegument leading to loss of adherence to host tissues ultimately causing disintegration and expulsion of parasites.

Praziquantel does exert its antiparasitic effects directly also. Level of durgs are increased if consumed with food (carbohydrate) or with cimetidine. There may be reduced serum levels of this drug by chloroquine, carbamazepine, phenytoid and also glucocorticoids, etc. In human the drug is completely metabolized and mostly excreted through urine.

Indications

- Clonorchiasis
- Cystecercosis
- Diphyllobothriasis
- Hymenolepsiasis
- Teniasis
- Opisthorchiasis
- Intestinal trematodes
- Paragonimiasis
- Schistosomiasis.

Side Effect

- Abdominal pain
- Diarrhea
- Dizziness
- Headache
- Malaise
- Fever
- Nausea
- Puritis.

Breast milk: It is present in breast milk.

PYRANTEL PAMATE

It is quite safe, well tolerated cheap indicated in intestinal nematodal infections. However, it is not effective in trichuriasis. It is effective and administered in single dose. It exerts its action on nematodes by depolarization of neuromuscular junction resulting in irreversible paralysis allowing expulsion of worms with the stools.

It is poorly absorbed from intestine. It carries minimal toxicity and can be administered orally. However, it is not given to pregnant women and children of less than 12 months age.

Indications

Ascariasis
Enterobiasis
Hookworm
Trichostrongyloidiasis.

Side Effects

- Gastrointestinal disorders
- Headache
- Dizziness
- Increased aminotransferases

Contraindication

- Pregnancy.

THIABENDAZOLE (MINTEZOL)

It is effective against most nematodes infecting humans. This drug is absorbed readily from gastrointestinal tract. It is administered after meals. It is extensibly metabolized in the liver before being excreted as glucoromide or sulfate conjugates of 5-hydroxythiabendazole mostly in urine.

Mechanism of its action is a not exactly known. Most likely it is by inhibition of polymerization of parasite B tubulin. The drug also inhibits enzyme fumarate reductase. This drug may suppress egg and larval production by some nematodes and also inhibit the development of eggs or larva passed in stool.

Indications

- Strongyloidiasis
- Cutaneous larva migrans
- Visceral larva and migrans.

Side Effects

- Anorexia
- Nausea
- Vomiting
- Diarrhea
- Drowsiness
- Giddiness
- Crystoluria
- Elevated aminotransferases
- Hepatitis
- Seizures
- Angioneurotic edema
- Tinnitus
- Stevens-Johnson syndrome

Contraindication

- Pregnancy.

TRICLABENDAZOLE (FASINEX)

May be used in paragonimiasis and all stages of *Fasciola hepatica*. The active sulfoxide metabolite of triclabendazole binds to fluke tubulin by assuming a unique non-planar configuration and disrupts microtubule based processes.

It is rapidly absorbed orally and undergo metabolism in liver. If given with food there is enhanced absorption and shortening of half-life of active metabolite. Treatment is given in one or two doses.

Indications

- Fasioliasis
- Paragonimiasis.

Side Effects

- Abdominal cramps
- Diarrhea
- Headache.

Breast Milk

Present in breast milk.

ANTHELMINTHIC DRUGS AT A GLANCE

Table 12.1: Treatment of Helminth infections

Cestodes	***Primary agents***	***Alternative agents***
Taenia saginata	Praziquantel as a single 10–25 mg/kg dose	Niclosamide
Taenia solium	Praziquantel as a single 10–25 mg/kg dose	Niclosamide
Echinococcus granulosus	Albendazole—400 mg twice daily, usually minimum of 3-6 months	Praziquantel
Cysticercosis	Albendazole—400 mg twice daily, usually for 8 days (8–30 days)	Praziquantel
Hymenolepis nana	Nitazoxanide as a single oral dose of 50 mg/kg or twice daily for 3 days	Praziquantel
Trematodes		
Paragonimus westermani	Praziquantel—75 mg/kg/day in three doses for 2 days	Bithionol
Clonorchis sinensis	Praziquantel—75 mg/kg/day in three doses for 1 day	Albendazole
Fasciola hepatica	Triclabendazole	Nitazoxanide

Contd...

Contd...

Cestodes	***Primary agents***	***Alternative agents***
Intestinal flukes	Praziquantel—75 mg/kg/day in three doses for 1 day	
Schistosomes	Praziquantel—40–60 mg/kg/day in 2–3 doses for one day	
Nematodes		
Ascaris lumbricoides	Albendazole—single 400 mg dose	Mebendazole, pyrantel Pamoate, nitazoxanide
Hookworm	Albendazole—single 400 mg dose	Mebendazole, pyrantel pamoate
Cutaneous larva migrans	Albendazole—400 mg daily for 3 days	Ivermectin, topical thiabendazole
Enterobius vermicularis	Albendazole—400 mg dose, repeat in 2 weeks	Mebendazole, pyrantel Pamoate
Strongyloides stercoralis	Ivermectin—200μg/kg daily for 1-2 doses	Thiabendazole, Albendazole
Toxocara species (visceral larva migrans)	Albendazole—400 mg bd for 5 days	Mebendazole
Trichuris trichiura	Albendazole—single 400 mg dose, Mebendazole—500 mg single dose, 100 mg bd for 3 days	Ivermectin, Nitazoxanide
Filariasis (Wuchereria bancrofti and *Brugia malayi)*	Diethylcarbamazine (upto 6 mg/kg/day in 3 doses for 14 days or single dose, with or without albendazole or ivermectin)	
Loa loa	Diethylcarbamazine (upto 9 mg/kg/day in 3 doses for 21 days with or without albendazole or ivermectin)	
Onchocerca volvulus	Ivermectin—single 150 μg/kg dose: repeat every 6–12 months until asymptomatic	

Newer Anthelmintics

Nitazoxanide[1]

It is a new 5-nitrothiazole derivative with broad spectrum activity against numerous intestinal protozoa, helminths and anaerobic bacteria. Its mechanism of action in helminths has not yet been determined. The main indication of use after discovery in US is for treatment of Cryptosporidium parvum in immunocompromised children.

Its anti-helminthic property is used against *Ascaris, Echinococcus, Fasciola hepatica,* Hookworms, *Hymenolepis nana, Taenia saginata* and *Trichuris trichiura.*

Dosage: Children (1-3 years)—100 mg bd for 3 days
Children (4-11 years)—200 mg bd for 3 days
Adults—500 mg bd for 3 days
Immunocompromised—1000 mg bd for 2-8 weeks.

Adverse effects: Though well tolerated may lead to mild GIT disturbance in 3-4%. Safety in pregnant and lactating females is not established.

ARTEMISININ DERIVATIVES (ARTEMETHUR, ARTESUNATE)

It is an active ingredient of the herb *Artemisia annua* and its semi synthetic derivatives are some of the most potent anti-malarials curently available. These derivatives have been shown to have preventive effects in *Schistosoma japonicum* infections in animal models by killing immature worms.[2,3] This action was confirmed in humans in randomised double blind placebo controlled trials in China, where the incidence and intensity of infection in endemic areas was reduced significantly.[4] But further work needs to be done in epidemiological and public health areas for its efficacy to be established.

REFERENCES

1. Murray PR, Baron EJ, Jorgensen JH, et al. Manual of Clinical Microbiology, 9th edn, vol.2, ch 150; 2228–29.
2. Xiao SH, You JQ, Yang YQ, et al. Experimental studies on early treatment of Schistosomal infection with artemethur. Southeast Asian J Trop Med Public Health 1995; 26:306–18.
3. Xiao SH, You JQ, Mei JY, et al. Preventive effect of artemethur in rabbits infected with Schistosoma japonicum cercariae. Acta Pharmacol Sin. 1998; 19:63–66.
4. Xiao SH, Booth M, Tanner M. The prophylactic effect of antemethur against *Schistosoma japonicum* infections. Parasitol Today 2000; 16:12–126.

Summary

Helminth means worm. They are multicellular, bilaterally symmetrical elongated, flat or round triploblastic. They are divisible into two phyla, i.e. Platyhelminthes and Nemathelminthes. Platyhelminthes contain two classes cestodes (*Echinococcus granulosus*, etc.) and trematodes (*Schistosoma haematobium*, etc.). Nemathelminthes include, roundworm, hookworms, threadworms, etc.

Top helminths according to WHO include *Ascaris lumbricoides*, Hookworms, *Trichuris trichiura*, Filarial worms and Schistosomes.

Two features of helminths are worth remembering:

1. They do not multiply in the human body.
2. Preparation of vaccine is difficult uptill now but research work is in progress.

The history of helminths and associated helminths infections has been fascinating and a subject of excitement in medicine. It is believed that primitive tribes in Sarawak and North Borne people were perhaps aware of round worm and tapeworms. There after with passage of time researchers gathered knowledge on different helminths like roundworm, hookworms, pinworms, tenias, etc. This work is going on with identification and clinical importance of newer helminths even today. Definitely with the advances in biochemistry and molecular biology there is creation of additional species and subspecies (current list of over 300 species) available.

Helminths diseases contribute to mortality, morbidity, malnutrition, growth retardation and of course diminished work capacity. Uprising AIDS cases and other immunosuppressive conditions opportunistic helminthic infection, e.g. strongyloidosis is attaining topmost position all over the world including developed areas.

The mode of infection of helminthic diseases may be contagious, soil, arthropods, snails and animal food (*Taenia solium, Taenia saginata*). Role of helminths in causing disease include intestinal obstruction (*Ascaris lumbricoides*), pressure effect (hydatid disease), lymphatic obstruction (*Wuchereria bancrofti*), trauma (hookworm), host reaction, tumor (*Schistosoma hematobium*) and so on.

The factors responsible for high prevelance of helmenthiasis are high population density, poor sanitation, deficient water sources, poor hygiene, poverty, etc. Almost one-third of world population is suffering from helminthic diseases. Food borne trematode infections may be caused by fasciola, opisthochis, clonorchis, fasciolopis, etc. Along with this, helminth involving eyes, heart, gynecology patients are underlined.

Also discussed briefly the role of helminths in causing emergencies. Abdominal pain and other associated symptoms are common in heavy intestinal nematodes like roundworms, hookworms. There may be association between anisakiasis and appendicitis.

Regarding intestinal helminths, trichinella also known by the name trichina worm and is the causative agent of trichinosis. The adult worm remains buried in the duodenum or

Jejunal mucosa. Its larvae encyst in the striated muscle of human, pig. It is one of the smallest nematode infecting the humans. Mode of human infection is by ingestion of raw meat infested with cysts of *Trichinella spiralis.* Man manifestations are pain abdomen, nausea, vomiting diarrhea, fever, fatal myocarditis, etc. Muscle biopsy, xenodiagnosis and skin test are important to establish diagnosis. Thiabendazole, pyrantel pamoate, etc. may be used to treat patients.

Trichuris trichiura another intestinal helminth is also called whip worm. It lives in cecum and appendix of humans. The adult worm lives upto 3 years. Female worm is oviparous. Eggs are barrel shaped with mucus plugs at each pole. Children suffer from chronic dysentery, rectal prolapse, blood diarrhea, etc. It may be treated with albendazole, mebendazole, oxantel, etc.

Strongyloides stercoralis (female) lives buried within mucosa of intestine particularly duodenum and jejunum. Humans are infected by penetration of filariform larvae the intact skin and then through blood stream reach lungs, crawl over epiglottis and finally swallowed down to small intestine. Here they develop into adult form. They may cause gastrointestinal bleeding, paralytic ileus, protein losing enteropathy, etc. Immunosuppressive patients must be scanned for this parasite because of danger of hyperinfection with this parasite. Thiabendazole is drug of choice to treat it.

Enterobius vermicularis is also called threadworm. It has cosmopolitan distribution. Adult worm inhabit in cecum, appendix and ascending colon. Perianal pruritus is the characteristic feature of enterobiasis. It may cause appenditis, nocturnal itching, vulvo-vaginitis, etc. Demonstration of egg from perianal region at night is done with the help of NIH swab.

Ascaris lumbricoides are also called roundworm. It is cosmopolitan with worldwide distribution. The adult worm reside in small intestine especially Jejunum of human. Adult worms may cause malnutrition, retardation of growth, obstruction of intestine tract, etc. *Ancylostoma duodenal* and *Necator americanus* are also called hookworm. Adult worm lives in small intestine. Clinical manifestation include maculopapular rash, cough, epigastric discomfort, pica, iron-deficiency anemia, etc. In case anemia is present must be treated first and then anthelminthic drug may be given.

Clonorchis sinensis is also called chinese liver fluke. It requires one definitive host and two intermediate hosts. The metacercariae are infective form of parasite. In man it causes inflammation, fibrosis of bile duct, etc.

Fasciolopsis buski a helminth of small intestine of human is largest trematode parasitizing humans. It is responsible for causing hemorrhages and ulcers in intestine. Death of patient may occur due to intestine obstruction and malnutrition. Another intestinal helminth is *Diphyllobothrium latum* also named fish tapeworm. The adult form of this parasite get attached to the wall of ileum causing imbalance between intrinsic and extrinsic factors of Castle. The result is pernicious anemia.

Hymenolepis nana also called dwarf tapeworm. It lives in lumen of upper three quarters of ileum of human. Adult worm measure 1 to 4 cm × 1 mm. Autoinfection is the major feature of this helminth and it happens in immunocompromised patients.

Among *Taenia saginata* and *Taenia solium* it is *Taenia solium* which is more pathogenic and much of concern these days. *Taenia solium* is responsible for causing cysticercus cellulosae which may cause, subcutaneous, nodules. The nodules may be seen in muscles too. They may involve anterior and vitreous chamber of eye. They may develop in brain causing seizures.

Somatic or tissue helminths include *Paragonimus westermani, Dracunculus medinensis, Fasciola hepatica, Schistosoma, Echinococcus, Wuchereria bancrofti, Brugia malayi, Loa loa* and *Onchocerca volvulus. Paragonimus westermani* also called oriental lung fluke are found in cystic cavities of the lungs usually in pairs. Over nine species are identified. In cases of hemoptysis apart from *Mycobacterium tuberculosis*, this parasite may be the cause. Another somatic helminths is liver fluke. In fact it is *Fasciola hepatica* living in biliary passages of liver in humans. Adult worm is leaf like with 10 years life span. It may cause obstructive Jaundia. *Dracunculus medinensis* is referred as fiery serpent in bible. It may produce blister commonly feet are involved between metatarsal bones. Many a time blister may appear on ankle. Because of effective preventive measures *Dracunculus medinensis* is declared eradicated from Pakistan since 1993 and India since 1997.

Animal helminths like *Ancylostoma braziliense*, etc., *Toxocara canis*, etc., may involve humans causing larva migrans. It may have manifestations like intense itching (cutaneous larva migrans), asthma, arthralgia, petitmal epilepsy unilateral, painless lesion of eye (Visceral larva migrans).

Schistosomiasis is caused by *schistosoma*. Several theories are suggested to explain the possible role of *Schistosoma hematobium* in causing malignancy of urinary bladder. Schistosoma mansoni also called Manson's blood fluke. Adult worms live in mesenteric vein of sigmoidorectal region and also branches of portal veins of liver. It causes Katayma fever especially in heavy infection. It may be responsible for lymphadenopathy, hepatosplenomegaly, eosinophilia, etc. *Schistosoma japonicum* also called oriental blood fluke usually found in radicles of superior mesenteric vein draining ileocecal junction, rectal plexus, etc. It may cause Katayama syndrome, periportal cirrhosis portal hypertension, gastrointestinal bleeding, etc.

Hydatid disease is caused by *Echinococcus granulosus* and *Echinococcus multilocularis*. The other name given to *Echinococcus granulosus* is *Taenia echinococcus*. It is commonly found all over the world in cattle and sheep raising areas.

Man barber larval form commonly in liver and lungs. Adult form of this parasite is seen in small intestine of dog and other canine animals. In man this parasite causes a disease called hydatid cyst. The hydatid cyst may be asymptomatic. In case of rupture of hydatid cyst, it may lead to allergic manifestations which may be fatal. For diagnosing Casoni's test and is commonly used serological tests are quite useful especially with the use of caprons arc five antigen. Toward treatment it is surgical excision of cyst which is accepted treatment.

On the other side *Echinococcus multilocularis* produce multilocular infiltrating lesions which may be mistaken as malignant tumor. It may spread as malignant tumor. It is most lethal of all helminthic infections of humans. The multilocular cysts in man are sterile.

Filariasis has been known since antiquity *Wuchereria bancrofti* (adult form) lives in lymphatics whereas sheathed microfilariae may be found in blood stream. In peripheral blood film microfilariae are demonstrated if blood is collected between 10 PM and 4 A.M. Man is definitive host whereas mosquitoes (Culex, Aedes or Anopheles) are intermediate hosts. Pathological features are because of lymphangitis and lymphadenitis. Important clinical features include filarial fever, lymphangitis, lymphadenitis, hydrocele, lymphedema, elephantiasis, etc. to Laboratory diagnosis techniques include DNA probes. *Brugia malayi* is almost similar to *Wuchereria bancrofti*. *Brugia malayi* rarely causes genitalia elephantiasis. *Loa loa* worm was extracted from the eye of Negress in West Indies in 1770. It completes life cycle in two hosts (man and mango fly). It produces calabar swelling, itching, erythema, fever, edema of eyelid, proptosis and conjunctival granulomata. *Onchocerca volvulus* completes its life cycle in two hosts, man and female black fly. It causes itching with secondary bacterial infection producing severe dermatitis called Sowda, loss of elastic fibres in skin (hanging gown), keratitis, optical atrophy and blindness.

Certain helminths are reported to be linked with oncogenesis. They are schistosome opisthorchis, chlonorchis, *Taenia solium*, etc. *Schistosoma hematobium* and *Opisthorchis viverrini* are associated with carcinoma urinary bladder and cholangiocarcinoma respectively, *clonorchis sinensis* with cholangiocarcinoma and so on. Various mechanisms responsible for this association are discussed.

Helminths responsible for nosocomial infections are *Enterobius vermicularis, Strongyloides stercoralis, Hymenolepis nana, Taenia solium*, etc. Within the hospital complex interaction between food service personnels and patients need attention. Food handlers are to be checked closely for harboring helminths. Helminths involved in gastrointestinal nosocomial infections may be *Hymenolepis nana* and *Taenia solium. Strongyloides stercoralis* may cause serious diseases in immunocompromised patients.

International travel to tropical areas has increased over past few decades. This has increased emerging helminthic diseases. Overall increase in number of pet owning households has been accompanied by shift in types of less traditional pets (birds, rabbits, reptiles, fish, etc.). This has led to sudden appearance of helminthic diseases. The rare newly emerging helminthic disorders are gnathostomiasis, oesophagostomiasis, capillariasis, anisakidosis, eosinophilic enteritis, baylisascariasis, angiostrongyliasis, etc.

Helminthic control measures are being run in full swing. As a result some helminths have been brought under control. Onchocerciasis is eliminated from parts of Kenya, Nile, East Africa by using insecticide DDT. Local antimosquito spray has eliminated lymphatic filariasis from Solomon. *Brugia malayi* is eliminated from Sri Lanka with the use of DEC. Helminthic vaccine is really a challenge superadded with multiple problems. Some helminthic vaccines are under trial, e.g. vaccines for hookworm disease, schistosomiasis and teniasis. Many human anthelminthic disease vaccines are underdevelopment, e.g. hydatid disease, *Onchocerca volvulus*, etc.

Toward treatment of helminthic diseases many drugs are used successfully. They are albendazole, ivermectin, diethylcarbamazine, mebendazole, metrifonate, niclosamide, oxamniquine, praziquantel, pyrantel pamoate, thiabendazole, triclabendazole, etc. Some newer anthelminthic are available, e.g. nitazoxanide artemisinin derivatives, etc.

Glossary

A

Accidental host	Host other than normal host harboring a parasite
Acoelomate	Having no body cavity between the body and internal organ, e.g. platyhelminthes

B

Bilateral symmetry	Animals body is divisible into two (right and left) along with their length
Brood capsule	Daughter cyst having developing scolices enclosing structure inside

C

Cercaria	The larva of trematode worms
Cervical alae	Wing like expansion of cuticle near mouth
Cilium	A hair like structure which may be used for locomotion
Cloacea	A common chamber getting digestive waste and urogenital products
Coelom	A body cavity in triphoblastic animals
Curacidium	Ciliated larval stage of *Diphyllobothrium latum*
Coracidium	A ciliated oncosphere of *Diphyllobothrium*
Corticated	Presence of outer mammillated albuminous Coating
Copulatory bursa	An umbrella like expansion the cuticle surrounding cloaca of the male nematode of certain species. It is supported by fleshy rays comparable with the ribs of umbrella
Cuticle	Surface covering present on adult nematodes
Cysticercoid	Scolex surrounded by bladder like cyst with or without fluid

D

Decorticated	Absence of outer, mammillated albuminous coating
Digenea	Class of parasites which include flukes are also known digenea
Diecious	Having male and female sex organ in different individual of the same species
Dorsal	Pertaining to the back or posterior part of body or organ
Dorsoventral	As in an axis from back to belly of animal body

E

Egg shell	The outer membrane enclosing the oncosphere with embryophore and yolk sac

Embryophore	The enveloping membrane surrounding the oncosphere
Endoparasite	An organism living in or on the internal organs of the host, e.g. intestinal worms

F

Filariform Larva	Infective, non-feeding larva

G

Gravid	Pregnant
Gynecophoric canal	A channel formed by infolding of lateral margins of the body of male behind ventral sucker for holding female during computation

H

Hexacanth embryo	Motile first larval stage of some tapeworm armed with three pairs of hooks also called oncosphere

M

Metacercaria	A cercaria (Juvenile fluke) that has lost tadpole like tail and has become encysted in second intermediate host
Metacercaria	The encysted cercaria without a tank, infective to definitive hosts
Miracidium	The first larval form of liver fluke, developing from egg as a minute, ciliated free swimming larva
Monoecious	Having male and female organs in same individual. It is also called hermaphrodite

N

Nematoda	Round, slender, unsegmented worm, e.g. roundworm

O

Operculum	Any lid or flap like covering may be present on the egg of fluke
Oviparous	Pertaining to an animal bearing young ones that hatch from eggs outside the mother's body
Ovoviviparous	Pertaining to an animal bearing young ones that hatch from eggs retain within mother's body

P

Platyhelminthes	A phylum of multicellular acoelomate animal called flatworms which are flattened dorsoventrally and are bilateral symmetrical, e.g. trematodes, cestodes
Pseudocoel	A "falso" fluid filled cavity, e.g. nematode. It is called false because it is not lined with mesoderm

R

Redia	The larval stage in the life cycle of trematode worms (flukes) which eventually develop into cercarium
Rhabditiform larva	First stage feeding larva which is not infective

Rostellum	Fleshy extension of the scolex of some tapeworms. It may not be armed with hooks

S

Schistosomulum	The growing worm of schistosomes in definitive host
Scolex	Head like structure on the anterior end of tapeworm
Spicule	It represents the accessory copulatory organ. It is rod like protrusible
Sporocyst	The second larval stage of trematode
Striated muscle	Muscle tissue having distinct banding pattern due to regular arrangement of actin and myosin proteins
Strobila	Body of tapeworm
Suckers	Cup-shaped structure on the scolex

T

Tegument	Outer surface of tapeworm and flukes

U

Unembryonale	Unfertilized

V

Vas deferens	Duct leading from testis to penis in mammal or to the exterior, the urogenital canal or cloaca in other animals
Ventral	Pertaining to front surface of an organism
Viscera	Internal organs in the body cavity

INDEX

Page numbers followed by *f* refer to figure and *t* refer to table